Technologic Innovations in Rhinology

Guest Editor

RAJ SINDWANI, MD

OTOLARYNGOLOGIC CLINICS OF NORTH AMERICA

www.oto.theclinics.com

October 2009 • Volume 42 • Number 5

SAUNDERS an imprint of ELSEVIER, Inc.

W.B. SAUNDERS COMPANY

A Division of Elsevier Inc.

1600 John F. Kennedy Boulevard ● Suite 1800 ● Philadelphia, Pennsylvania 19103-2899

http://www.theclinics.com

OTOLARYNGOLOGIC CLINICS OF NORTH AMERICA Volume 42, Number 5
October 2009 ISSN 0030-6665, ISBN-13: 978-1-4377-1255-1, ISBN-10: 1-4377-1255-X

Editor: Joanne Husovski
Development Editor: Theresa Collier

Otolaryngologic Clinics of North America (ISSN 0030-6665) is published bimonthly by Elsevier, Inc., 360 Park Avenue South, New York, NY 10010-1710. Months of issue are February, April, June, August, October, and December. Business and Editorial Offices: 1600 John F. Kennedy Blvd., Suite 1800, Philadelphia, PA 19103-2899. Customer Service Office: 6277 Sea Harbor Drive, Orlando, FL 32887-4800. Periodicals postage paid at New York, NY and additional mailing offices. Subscription prices is $264.00 per year (US individuals), $488.00 per year (US institutions), $129.00 per year (US student/resident), $347.00 per year (Canadian individuals), $613.00 per year (Canadian institutions), $390.00 per year (international individuals), $613.00 per year (international institutions), $199.00 per year (international & Canadian student/resident). Foreign air speed delivery is included in all *Clinics'* subscription prices. All prices are subject to change without notice. **POSTMASTER:** Send address changes to *Otolaryngologic Clinics of North America*, Elsevier Health Sciences Division, Subscription Customer Service, 3251 Riverport Lane, Maryland Heights, MO 63043. **Telephone: 1-800-654-2452 (U.S. and Canada); 314-447-8871 (outside U.S. and Canada). Fax: 314-447-8029. E-mail: journalscustomerservice-usa@elsevier.com (for print support); journalsonlinesupport-usa@elsevier.com (for online support).**

Reprints. For copies of 100 or more of articles in this publication, please contact the Commercial Reprints Department, Elsevier Inc., 360 Park Avenue South, New York, NY 10010-1710. Tel.: 212-633-3812; Fax: 212-462-1935; E-mail: reprints@elsevier.com.

Otolaryngologic Clinics of North America is also published in Spanish by McGraw-Hill Interamericana Editores S.A., P.O. Box 5-237, 06500 Mexico D.F., Mexico.

Otolaryngologic Clinics of North America is covered in *MEDLINE/PubMed (Index Medicus), Current Contents/Clinical Medicine, Excerpta Medica, BIOSIS, Science Citation Index,* and *ISI/BIOMED.*

Printed and bound by CPI Group (UK) Ltd, Croydon, CR0 4YY

Transferred to Digital Print 2011

Contributors

GUEST EDITOR

RAJ SINDWANI, MD, FACS, FRCS(C)
Associate Professor of Otolaryngology, Department of Otolaryngology–Head & Neck Surgery, Division of Rhinology & Sinus Surgery, St Louis University School of Medicine, St Louis, Missouri

AUTHORS

NAFI AYGUN, MD
The Russell H. Morgan Department of Radiology and Radiological Sciences, The Johns Hopkins Medical Institutions, Baltimore, Maryland

KAREN A. BEDNARSKI, MD
Georgia Nasal and Sinus Institute, Savannah, Georgia

BENJAMIN S. BLEIER, MD
Department of Otorhinolaryngology–Head and Neck Surgery, University of Pennsylvania School of Medicine, Villanova, Philadelphia, Pennsylvania

SETH BRUGGERS, MD
Resident, Department of Otolaryngology–Head & Neck Surgery, St Louis University School of Medicine, St Louis, Missouri

PAUL D. CAMPBELL, Jr, MD
The Russell H. Morgan Department of Radiology and Radiological Sciences, The Johns Hopkins Medical Institutions, Baltimore, Maryland

RICARDO L. CARRAU, MD
Department of Otolaryngology–Head and Neck Surgery, University of Pittsburgh School of Medicine, Pittsburgh, Pennsylvania; Department of Neurosurgery, University of Pittsburgh School of Medicine, Pittsburgh, Pennsylvania

RAKESH K. CHANDRA, MD
Associate Professor, Northwestern Sinus & Allergy Center, Department of Otolaryngology–Head & Neck Surgery, Northwestern University Feinberg School of Medicine, Chicago, Illinois

MARTIN J. CITARDI, MD
Professor, Department of Otorhinolaryngology–Head and Neck Surgery, University of Texas Medical School at Houston, Texas Sinus Institute, Texas Skull Base Institute, Houston, Texas

DAVID B. CONLEY, MD
Associate Professor, Northwestern Sinus & Allergy Center, Department of Otolaryngology–Head & Neck Surgery, Northwestern University Feinberg School of Medicine, Chicago, Illinois

DARY J. COSTA, MD
Department of Otolaryngology–Head & Neck Surgery, St Louis University School of Medicine, St Louis, Missouri

JEFFREY L. CUTLER, MD
Assistant Professor, Uniform Services University of the Health Sciences; Director of Rhinology, Nasal Sinus Surgery, Department of Surgery, Section of Otolaryngology, Head and Neck Surgery, Walter Reed Army Medical Center, NW, Washington, DC

SAMER FAKHRI, MD
Associate Professor, Department of Otorhinolaryngology–Head and Neck Surgery, University of Texas Medical School at Houston, Texas Sinus Institute, Texas Skull Base Institute, Houston, Texas

MARVIN P. FRIED, MD
Professor and University Chairman, Department of Otorhinolaryngology–Head and Neck Surgery, Montefiore Medical Center, Bronx, New York

PAUL GARDNER, MD
Department of Neurosurgery, University of Pittsburgh School of Medicine, Pittsburgh, Pennsylvania

MARC GIBBER, MD
Surgical Resident, Department of Otorhinolaryngology–Head and Neck Surgery, Montefiore Medical Center, Bronx, New York

RICHARD J. HARVEY, MD
Senior Lecturer, Rhinology and Skull Base Surgery, Department of Otolaryngology/Skull Base Surgery, St Vincent's Hospital, Darlinghurst, Sydney, NSW, Australia

SETH ISAACS, MD
Fellow, Department of Otorhinolaryngology–Head and Neck Surgery, University of Texas Medical School at Houston, Texas Sinus Institute, Texas Skull Base Institute, Houston, Texas

AMIN B. KASSAM, MD
St John's Health Center, John Wayne Cancer Institute, Santa Monica, California

RACHEL KAYE, BA
Candidate for Medical Doctorate, Albert Einstein College of Medicine, Bronx, New York

ROBERT C. KERN, MD
Professor, Northwestern Sinus & Allergy Center, Department of Otolaryngology–Head & Neck Surgery, Northwestern University Feinberg School of Medicine, Chicago, Illinois

ESTHER KIM, MD
Department of Surgery, Section of Otolaryngology, Head and Neck Surgery, Walter Reed Army Medical Center, NW, Washington, DC

FREDERICK A. KUHN, MD, FACS
Director Georgia Nasal and Sinus Institute, Savannah, Georgia; Associate Professor, Department of Otolaryngology–Head and Neck Surgery, University of North Carolina at Chapel Hill, Chapel Hill, North Carolina

ANDREW P. LANE, MD
Associate Professor and Director, Division of Rhinology and Sinus Surgery, Department of Otolaryngology–Head and Neck Surgery, The Johns Hopkins School of Medicine, Baltimore, Maryland

AMBER LUONG, MD, PhD
Assistant Professor, Department of Otorhinolaryngology–Head and Neck Surgery, University of Texas Medical School at Houston, Texas Sinus Institute, Texas Skull Base Institute, Houston, Texas

BRADLEY F. MARPLE, MD
Professor and Vice Chair, Department of Otolaryngology–Head and Neck Surgery, University of Texas, Southwestern Medical Center, Dallas, Texas

RICHARD R. ORLANDI, MD
Associate Professor, Division of Otolaryngology–Head and Neck Surgery, University of Utah, Salt Lake City, Utah; Associate Director, Center for Therapeutic Biomaterials, University of Utah, Salt Lake City, Utah

JAMES N. PALMER, MD
Associate Professor, Director, Division of Rhinology, Department of Otorhinolaryngology–Head and Neck Surgery, University of Pennsylvania School of Medicine, Philadelphia, Pennsylvania

DANIEL M. PREVEDELLO, MD
Department of Neurosurgery, University of Pittsburgh School of Medicine, Pittsburgh, Pennsylvania

MURUGAPPAN RAMANATHAN, Jr, MD
Fellow, Division of Rhinology and Sinus Surgery, Department of Otolaryngology–Head and Neck Surgery, The Johns Hopkins School of Medicine, Baltimore, Maryland

RODNEY J. SCHLOSSER, MD
Professor and Director of Rhinology and Skull Base Surgery, Department of Otolaryngology/Head & Neck Surgery, Medical University of South Carolina, Charleston, South Carolina

RAJ SINDWANI, MD, FACS, FRCS(C)
Associate Professor of Otolaryngology, Department of Otolaryngology–Head & Neck Surgery, Division of Rhinology & Sinus Surgery, St Louis University School of Medicine, St Louis, Missouri

CARL H. SNYDERMAN, MD
Department of Otolaryngology–Head and Neck Surgery, University of Pittsburgh School of Medicine, Pittsburgh, Pennsylvania; Department of Neurosurgery, University of Pittsburgh School of Medicine, Pittsburgh, Pennsylvania

JUSTIN H. TURNER, MD, PhD
Resident, Department of Otolaryngology–Head and Neck Surgery, The Johns Hopkins School of Medicine, Baltimore, Maryland

ROWAN VALENTINE, MBBS
Department of Surgery-Otorhinolaryngology, Head and Neck Surgery, The Queen Elizabeth Hospital, University of Adelaide, Woodville, Adelaide, South Australia, Australia

PETER-JOHN WORMALD, MD
Department of Surgery-Otorhinolaryngology, Head and Neck Surgery,
The Queen Elizabeth Hospital, University of Adelaide, Woodville, Adelaide,
South Australia, Australia

S. JAMES ZINREICH, MD
The Russell H. Morgan Department of Radiology and Radiological Sciences,
The Johns Hopkins Medical Institutions, Baltimore, Maryland

Contents

New technologies continue to affect the practice of otolaryngology–head and neck surgery. Numerous financial and regulatory barriers must be overcome to develop an idea into a useful device or intervention. US Food and Drug Administration (FDA) approval focuses on safety, often leaving the medical community, in general, to determine the efficacy of the device after FDA approval has been granted. Physicians are involved throughout the technology development process, generating conflicts of interest that must be effectively managed. It is essential that physicians ethically maintain their leadership in developing and evaluating new advances in medical technology.

Advances in instrumentation are part of the natural evolution of any surgical discipline. During this process, there are certain key junctures where the state of the art in technology truly augments the surgeon's ability to manage higher levels of pathology. The present era of endoscopic sinus surgery has been hallmarked by extension of minimally invasive techniques to complex pathologies including advanced inflammatory disease, and pathology involving the orbit, skull base, and brain. Evolution of the armamentarium for endoscopic visualization has been a central feature in this. In this article, key historical elements are reviewed and the technical principles behind these important advances in endoscopic visualization are discussed.

Since the introduction of functional endoscopic sinus surgery (FESS) in the United States in 1985, the information gained from imaging has proved imperative in understanding regional morphology and guidance of surgical procedures. More than 20 years later, the importance of imaging continues to be the anatomic detail afforded by this technology, the roadmap it provides in planning the surgery, and the morphologic detail it provides in recurrent disease. The latest development in CT technology, cone beam CT instrumentation, may change the way imaging of the nasal cavity and paranasal sinuses is performed in the future. These topics are discussed in this article.

Surgical navigation technology provides real-time intraoperative localization of surgical instruments within the field. These systems are highly accurate, assist with preoperative planning, and improve surgeon confidence. The industry has recently responded to the growing trend of treatment in ambulatory surgical centers by offering surgical navigation devices that are more compact, less expensive and more user-friendly than conventional devices. Surgical navigation is indicated for complex sinonasal disease and may reduce the risk of complications. The indications for surgical navigation continue to expand as the technology improves and imaging data synthesis evolves to include multimodality fusion and real-time intraoperative data-set updates. Although now widely available, navigation systems are still considered state of the art, and not standard of care.

Absorbable biomaterials are commonly used after endoscopic sinus surgery, both for hemostatic and wound healing considerations. Although removable nasal packing is the traditional method of controlling ongoing bleeding and modulating wound healing, it is uncomfortable for patients and associated with several complications. Currently available absorbable agents frequently incite an inflammatory reaction and have been shown in animal and human trials to adversely affect the wound healing process. Newer agents offer distinct advantages because of their unique composition and rapid clearance profiles. The selection of packing material used in any given sinus procedure should be based on surgeon preference and the details of the specific case.

Topical drug delivery for sinonasal disorders is influenced by a variety of factors. Macroscopically (or anatomically), the ability of the drug to reach the appropriate region of the paranasal system is paramount. Delivery techniques, surgical state of the sinus cavity, delivery device, and fluid dynamics (volume, pressure, position) have a significant impact on the delivery of topical therapies to the sinus mucosa. Once topical therapeutics actually reach the desired site, factors within the local microenvironment heavily influence local drug delivery. The presence and composition of the mucus blanket, mucociliary clearance, direct mucin-drug binding, and the permeability of pharmaceutical compounds will all impact drug delivery. In addition, the general therapeutic goal of topical management may lie between the potentially competing actions of mechanical lavage and pharmaceutical intervention. Techniques for the mechanical removal of mucus, antigen, and inflammatory products may not be the most efficient approach for pharmaceutical delivery. This article reviews the evolving concepts in local drug therapy, both for the factors that influence anatomic distribution within the sinonasal system and those that affect mucosal absorption.

Marc Gibber, Rachel Kaye, and Marvin P. Fried

Surgical simulation technology has advanced significantly in recent years. Medical-simulation validation studies have established that surgical skills honed using a simulator significantly improved trainee performance by decreasing operating times, improving efficiency, and decreasing errors. Integration of surgical simulation technologies into the medical training and education system improves the quality of the graduating surgeon, reduces the time to proficiency, and improves overall patient safety. This article discusses the current state of medical-simulator technology research, development, and use. It points to growing support from the surgical governing and regulation agencies; and predicts that medical students and surgical residents will be able, and mandated, to develop procedural skills in a life-like and no-risk environment.

Benjamin S. Bleier and James N. Palmer

As the scope of transnasal cranial-base surgery expands, reconstruction of the complex residual defects remains a challenge. Laser welding is a novel technology that can be performed endoscopically and offers the potential of producing instantaneous, watertight repairs using a chromophore-doped biologic solder.

THE CLINICS ARE NOW AVAILABLE ONLINE!

Access your subscription at:
www.theclinics.com

Preface

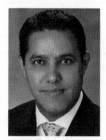

Raj Sindwani, MD, FACS, FRCS(C)
Guest Editor

Techniques in endoscopic sinus and skull base surgery have continued to evolve, often propelled forward by technological innovations. The introduction of the rigid nasal endoscope to the diagnosis and surgical management of sinonasal disorders is undeniably the single greatest advance in the field of rhinology to date. Rigid nasal endoscopy provided improved visualization of sinonasal anatomy and ushered in minimally invasive techniques of functionally oriented sinus surgery. Emboldened by the later application of powered microdebriders, drills, and surgical navigations systems, rhinologists continued to refine their endoscopic skills and began to follow disease processes that extended outside of the confines of the sinonasal tract. This evolution has led endoscopic surgeons to greatly expand their repertoires to safely and confidently address more complex pathologies involving the orbit, skull base, and even brain.

Technology plays a major role in all aspects of medicine and surgery, but few disciplines have been as robustly affected by technological advances as the field of rhinology. The reasons for this are likely multiple: a wide surgical audience that performs procedures for a very common, incurable problem that has a significant impact on quality of life; a relatively young technology-savvy specialty that actually redefined itself based on a technological innovation; and the backdrop of a larger movement across all areas of surgery to become "minimally invasive." Industry was watching— and it still is.

This collection of articles explores the technical workings, clinical applications, and impact on outcomes of the use of recent technological innovations in endoscopic sinus surgery. The leading experts who have kindly contributed to this effort have been charged with frankly commenting upon the current limitations and advantages of these new tools, and to project what future modifications may follow. We have also included an in-depth discussion of the current processes that device developers are required to negotiate to obtain Food and Drug Administration clearance before their instruments can be integrated into our operating rooms. As mentioned, *industry is watching—* and our relations with the companies that develop and market the tools that enable us are sensitive, highly complex, and under increasing scrutiny.

Otolaryngol Clin N Am 42 (2009) xiii–xv
doi:10.1016/j.otc.2009.08.020
0030-6665/09/$ – see front matter © 2009 Elsevier Inc. All rights reserved.

Like the endoscope, microdebrider, and the surgical navigation system, which have left an indelible mark on the face of rhinologic surgery, the innovations highlighted in this resource may also one day, as we venture toward new horizons, become mainstays in the endoscopic surgeon's armamentarium.

Raj Sindwani, MD, FACS, FRCS(C)
Department of Otolaryngology-Head & Neck Surgery
Division of Rhinology & Sinus Surgery
St Louis University School of Medicine
St Louis, MO, USA

E-mail address:
Sindwani@slu.edu

DEDICATION

To my girls,
Raj Sindwani

Developing, Regulating, and Ethically Evaluating New Technologies in Otolaryngology–Head and Neck Surgery

Richard R. Orlandi, MD[a,b,*], Bradley F. Marple, MD[c]

KEYWORDS

- Device • Technology • Regulatory approval
- Conflict of interest • Disclosure

Technology has always been a part of the practice of medicine. Stethoscopes and sphygmomanometers were as revolutionary a change when they were developed as advanced imaging or minimally invasive surgical techniques have been more recently. Physicians are driven to provide the best possible care for their patients, which often leads to the development, evaluation, and adoption of new medical technologies. This phenomenon is seen in otolaryngology–head and neck surgery, where diagnostic or therapeutic advances can make disease processes more accessible (eg, endoscopy) or allow them to be treated with less morbidity (eg, microscopic surgical advances in laryngology).

Integration of a new technology in medicine would ideally be preceded by a rigorous objective evaluation of safety and efficacy. An underpinning of evidence-based

---

Disclosures: Dr Orlandi, Stockholder and consultant: Carbylan BioSurgery, Inc, Consultant: Entellus Medical, Inc; Dr Marple, Consultant: Alcon, Medtronic, Speaker's bureau: Sepracor, Stockholder: Novabay. Funding: None.

[a] Division of Otolaryngology–Head and Neck Surgery, University of Utah, 50 North Medical Drive, 3C120, Salt Lake City, UT 84132, USA

[b] Center for Therapeutic Biomaterials, University of Utah, 50 North Medical Drive, 3C120, Salt Lake City, UT 84132, USA

[c] Department of Otolaryngology–Head and Neck Surgery, University of Texas, Southwestern Medical Center, 5323 Harry Hines Boulevard, Dallas, TX 75390-9035, USA

* Corresponding author. Division of Otolaryngology–Head and Neck Surgery, University of Utah, 50 North Medical Drive, 3C120, Salt Lake City, UT 84132.

E-mail address: richard.orlandi@hsc.utah.edu (R.R. Orlandi).

doi:10.1016/j.otc.2009.07.007
0030-6665/09/$ – see front matter
oto.theclinics.com

medicine (EBM) is that physicians provide the best care for their patients when it is based on such objective evidence. With regard to new technologic advances, however, practicing strict EBM is often not practical. Medical device developers are subject to numerous financial pressures that require them to bring their products to market and facilitate their use before efficacy is rigorously demonstrated. Moreover, current device regulation takes a rather permissive approach, with most developers using an approval mechanism that compares novel devices to currently approved products.

Rhinology, which has arguably undergone revolutionary changes in the last 20 years, provides multiple examples of generalized adoption of technology preceding evidence of efficacy, often by several years. Endoscopic sinus surgery was first practiced in the United States in the early 1980s, having been adopted from practices in Europe. The first widely published report of the technique appeared in the United States in 1985, followed by a generalized adoption of this technique during the ensuing decade.[1] It is instructive to point out, however, that evidence of efficacy of this new technique did not appear until the early 1990s.[2–4] Powered instrumentation is another technique that has significantly affected rhinology, whereby its description and adoption preceded evidence of its efficacy by about 5 years.[5,6] Image guidance has made an increasing impact on rhinology, going from a technology limited to tertiary rhinology practices to a tool available to most rhinologic surgeons.[7,8] Nevertheless, the evidence supporting its use in endoscopic sinus procedures is limited.[8,9] These examples illustrate that despite physicians' dedication to the principles of EBM, valuable new technologies are often adopted before the demonstration of their efficacy.

DEVELOPING AN IDEA INTO A MEDICAL DEVICE

A new device is invented by a physician and/or an engineer responding to an unmet clinical need. The inventor (or his or her employer, particularly in an academic setting) thus becomes the owner of intellectual property (IP), which is usually protected by patenting the invention. This process typically costs $5000 to $10,000, a cost borne by the owner of the IP. This cost is in addition to any development costs in materials or time that the inventor has already expended. The next step is to develop the invention into a mass-producible and mass-useable device. This is another time- and investment-intensive process, whereby the physician-inventor either partners with or becomes an entrepreneur, a person who strongly believes in the potential of the investment and is accustomed to high risk, hoping for what is often a long-delayed future reward. Indeed, it has been suggested that the definition of an entrepreneur is an individual willing to work very hard for free.

As the device is further refined, a final product eventually results. The final steps in this process must be performed using regulated Good Manufacturing Practices and Good Laboratory Practices, known separately as GMP and GLP. Toxicity measurements must also be performed according to international standards. These methods are necessary to satisfy the regulations that govern devices in the United States and Europe. The processes necessary to bring a device to practice are obviously beyond the capabilities of a physician's basement workshop. The development of a medical device from idea to final product thus requires between 10 and 20 million dollars.[10] These extensive financial resources are often supplied by a venture capital group, and increased risks are adopted in the hopes of increased potential returns on that investment. Alternatively, an established medical device company may partner with the physician-inventor, expending similar resources and expecting a similar return for that investment.

OBTAINING FDA APPROVAL

Medical devices in the United States are regulated by the Center for Devices and Radiological Health (CDRH) of the FDA, a branch of the Department of Health and Human Services. The FDA's drug-regulation and device-regulation mandates have evolved separately, so that these 2 classes are regulated differently. The Food and Drug Act of 1906 established the FDA's legal basis for regulation. The Federal Food, Drug, and Cosmetic Act of 1938 required the FDA to establish the safety of drugs, and it was not until the Kefauver-Harris Drug Amendments of 1962 that proof of drug effectiveness was required. It was not until 1976 that medical devices were specifically addressed by the Congress. The Medical Device Amendments of 1976 expanded the FDA's role in device regulation and specifically required the CDRH to assign devices into 1 of 3 classes, based on their complexity and potential risk and thus their need for regulation.[11]

The scope of medical devices is staggering. The CDRH regulates nearly 2000 types of devices, ranging from bandages and gloves to pacemakers and tissue allografts. Of these nearly 2000 types of devices, about 500,000 medical device models from 23,000 different manufacturers are monitored by the CDRH. Medical devices affect the care of nearly every patient in the United States, with 4% of patients having an implanted device. Medical devices comprise a 130-billion-dollar industry worldwide, with nearly half of the consumption taking place in the United States.[12] The FDA's device-approval process is divided into 2 pathways, depending on the degree of novelty and risk of the proposed device.[13]

Approval for a novel or high-risk device may start with an application for Premarket Approval (PMA), and the process is similar to the review of a new drug. The PMA review process requires clinical evidence of safety and efficacy before approval. Because of the increased time and expense of this more rigorous process, less than 100 of the approximately 4000 applications that the FDA receives each year are PMAs.[12]

The second, more streamlined process available for devices is known as the 510(k) pathway. This process is used when the proposed device can be demonstrated to be "substantially equivalent" to a device that already has FDA approval. In this context, the previously approved device is known as a predicate device. This process is much quicker, with approval occurring within 90 days of application submission, typically without a requirement for clinical evidence of efficacy. In fact, 90% of 510(k) applications have no such clinical data submitted. With more than 95% of medical devices receiving FDA approval as a result of this expedited 510(k) process, most devices reaching the physician's hands have not objectively demonstrated clinical efficacy. The current regulatory environment thus facilitates the availability of the latest potential clinical advances for patients. This "buyer beware" arrangement implicitly relies on individual practitioners to determine, often based on scant evidence, whether a device is most likely to be beneficial to an individual patient or not. It leaves proof of efficacy to practitioners rather than tying up potential advances in prolonged regulatory processes. In fact, it is during this postmarketing phase that evidence of efficacy is developed (and additional safety data is accumulated). For this reason, medical technologies enter clinical use well before their efficacy is established.

OBTAINING THIRD PARTY PAYER COVERAGE

Barriers to widespread adoption, nevertheless, do exist in the form of reimbursement regulations. The Centers for Medicare and Medicaid Services (CMS) originated in 1965 as part of the Social Security Administration and in 1977 became the Health Care

Financing Administration (HCFA). Renamed in 2001, CMS continues the original charge in its founding legislation, which mandates that diagnostic and treatment interventions must be determined to be "reasonable and necessary" for them to be reimbursed. Payment for the use of a device has an enormous impact on its adoption inasmuch as many third party payers follow CMS's policies, so that at some point, efficacy must be established for a manufacturer to have a sustainable market. Interestingly, CMS coverage decisions are usually not made centrally but rather are based on Local Medical Review Policies (LMRPs). LMRPs are issued by local Medicare carriers, which are advised by a Carrier Advisory Committee (CAC) composed of physicians from various specialties. The CAC partners with the carrier to evaluate existing medical evidence and provides input into coverage decisions. One local carrier's LMRP is often adopted by other carriers. Central policy decisions are made by CMS very rarely, usually when local LMRPs conflict, and these decisions are called National Coverage Decisions.

Occasionally, a new device is such an advance that it results in a new procedure. When this occurs, the manufacturer faces another hurdle for reimbursement, that is, development of a new procedural code. The Current Procedural Terminology (CPT) system was first developed in 1966 by the American Medical Association (AMA), and it was adopted by HCFA in 1986 as part of its Healthcare Common Procedure Coding System. CPT codes are maintained by the CPT Editorial Panel of the AMA, made up of 17 physicians and advised by the CPT Advisory Committee, which is made up of representatives from each national medical specialty society seated in the AMA House of Delegates. Otolaryngologists are represented by the American Academy of Otolaryngology–Head and Neck Surgery delegate.

New CPT codes and edits of existing CPT codes can be requested, with the request typically (but not necessarily) channeled through the specialty society (or, in some cases, societies) affected by the new procedure. These requests require clinical vignettes that illustrate the typical procedure and the proposed use of the medical device. The AMA has a series of established requirements, all of which must be met for the approval of a new or revised CPT code[14]:

First, the new devices to be used in the procedure must have received approval from the FDA for the specific use proposed.

Second, the procedure must be performed by many physicians or practitioners across the United States.

Third, the clinical efficacy of the procedure must be well established and documented in US peer review literature.

Fourth, the procedure can neither be a fragmentation of an existing procedure nor be currently reportable by 1 or more existing codes.

Fifth, the procedure cannot be requested as a means to report extraordinary circumstances related to the performance of a procedure already having a specific CPT code.

New devices, especially those that generate associated new procedures requiring new CPT codes, face an uphill battle for reimbursement without third party payer approval. New device distributors must often walk the fine line between touting the device's advances over what is currently available and appearing so new or revolutionary that additional regulatory interventions are needed. When a new device crosses this line into the area of a new procedure, the return on the inventors', entrepreneurs', and venture capitalists' investment can be substantially delayed inasmuch as a new CPT code requires proof of efficacy, which follows rather than precedes entry into the medical market, often by years. This fact can leave manufacturers and their investors substantially pressured to develop an early substantial revenue stream to see the device through the lag between FDA and CMS (and AMA) approval. Direct-to-consumer advertising and lay-press reporting of the purported medical advance associated with the device often is the result.

ETHICAL EVALUATION AND ADOPTION OF NEW TECHNOLOGIES

The development, evaluation, and adoption of a new medical device generate a clash of multiple interests. Conflicts of interest (COIs) involving physicians are inherent in taking a new technology from idea to the bedside. Impossible to avoid, these conflicts must instead be managed. The entrepreneurial forces of device development, by their very nature, push a device's entry into clinical practice as early and as rapidly as possible. This is necessitated by the realities of venture capital, where a rapid and large return on investment is desirable and is a part of the investment contract. Most agreements for venture investments mandate a multiple-fold return when the startup company is sold or acquired, before the original inventor or entrepreneur receives any proceeds from that sale or acquisition.

This arrangement creates a further conflict for the physician or scientist or inventor. Physicians are trained in the scientific method, whereby an advance is disseminated and verified by objective outside experts. Protection of IP and return on venture capital investments make this method impractical and nearly impossible. The physician who conceived of a true advance that will benefit patients must therefore usually make compromises to get that advance into the hands of practitioners, where it will indeed provide patient benefit. Moreover, the business forces that encourage rapid entry of the device into the market (even if it is not completely tested) may include the physician-inventor to some degree, in that he or she has invested significant time and financial resources in the early stages of the device development. Physician-inventors have a vested interest in recouping a return on this investment during early device development. The pressure to "get to market" and the return on investment that such market entry entails creates another conflict for the physician-inventor.

Other physicians may develop COIs as device development moves into a commercial setting. At this stage, companies will often identify respected leaders in academic medicine and private practice, referred to as "key opinion leaders" (KOLs), in the new technology's targeted medical field. Opinions from these KOLs are often sought in determining development strategies and in other decisions, such as packaging and marketing and in the development of clinical trials (whether pre- or postmarketing). The guidance provided by KOLs in the medical community is crucial to the optimal development of a useful new technology that can benefit patients, and to prove its efficacy. It is therefore not only tolerable or appropriate but also absolutely necessary for physicians to be involved in this process.

Physician involvement in new technology development is typically compensated, yet many startup companies and entrepreneurs have very little cash. These economic realities mean that physician consultants are often offered equity in the company in exchange for their services, either in combination with monetary payments or in lieu of them. The physician consultant will then have an interest in seeing the technology succeed, to increase the value of the stock holding. Even without a stock position, continued receipt of consulting fees relies upon continued success of the company and its product(s). This arrangement has the potential to affect his or her interpretation or presentation of data about the new technology. For example, it is preferred that clinical trials exclude or limit the involvement of clinicians who have a vested interest in seeing the technology succeed, potentially putting the physician's or investigator's interests at odds with those of the patient or subject. Regulatory approval can also be affected by these conflicts because data relative to safety and efficacy are often generated by physicians who are involved in the early stages of the device development and thus are potentially conflicted.

In any case, participation with any company should be plainly and prominently disclosed. Standards set by continuing education accreditation associations and journal editorial boards should be seen as a minimum. It is incumbent on any speaker or writer to do everything in his or her power to make sure the listener or reader is aware of any potential COI. Presentations in the lay press or discussions with patients about proposed early use of an unproven device are other areas where explicit disclosure is appropriate. In this way, the presented information can be interpreted in the context of any potential bias.

Early use of a new technology may occur with the intention of systematically collecting data about its efficacy, typically but not always in conjunction with the developer or distributor of the device. Such use satisfies the definition of research on human subjects and, therefore, must be overseen by an institutional review board, as required by multiple federal regulations and ethical standards.[15,16]

All of these factors must be taken into account as a physician evaluates a new technology and determines whether to use it to benefit a particular patient. The physician must remember that FDA approval likely says little about the device's efficacy. As a result of direct-to-consumer advertising, patients may request or even demand that a new device or procedure be used to remedy their condition. It is incumbent on the physician to be fully informed about the device or procedure specifically and about the device-development process in general as he or she evaluates the potential benefits and risks to patients, including inefficacy and increased expense.

Patients look to physicians to provide accurate information about treatment options, and the public looks to physicians to interpret new advances in medicine. New technologies should not be shunned a priori until high-level evidence is available, as this can take years. The ethics of embracing a potentially ineffective technology must be balanced with the ethics of denying patients a potential significant advance. The challenge will always lie in determining the point at which a significant benefit of a new technology can be reasonably assumed while maintaining a posture of academic vigilance that stimulates ongoing study. Continued pressure by the medical profession is needed to ensure that appropriate unbiased data regarding new technology help to refine our knowledge base as it relates to technique, indications, patient safety, and economics.

SUMMARY

New technologies affect otolaryngology–head and neck surgery and medicine in general and likely will continue to do so as long as physicians treat patients. The FDA approval process currently allows devices with unproven efficacy to be marketed; yet CMS and other third party payers significantly affect the adoption of these technologies by regulating their reimbursement. Development of a device-associated new procedure by the AMA can further affect the adoption of a new technology. Notwithstanding these hurdles, physicians must be aware that FDA-approved devices do not yet have systematically established efficacy, and they should include this information in their informed consent process with patients, especially when payment for the device may not be reimbursed by the patient's third party payer.

The process of taking a device from concept to bedside is an arduous and expensive one, necessitating the physician's or inventor's dogged determination and, commonly, an infusion of financial investment. Necessary involvement of business interests in the development of a device to be used by physicians to benefit patients unavoidably generates COIs. These inherent COIs should be managed, primarily through energetic full disclosure. It is appropriate and essential that physicians are involved with the process of technology development. Physicians should involve themselves in new technology development in spite of potential conflicts and should ethically manage those inherent conflicts. Continued advances in medicine rely on physicians to maintain their leadership role in continuing to develop and then to carefully evaluate new technologies.

REFERENCES

1. Kennedy DW. Functional endoscopic sinus surgery. Technique. Arch Otolaryngol 1985;111(10):643–9.
2. Hoffman SR, Mahoney MC, Chmiel JF, et al. Symptom relief after endoscopic sinus surgery: an outcomes-based study. Ear Nose Throat J 1993;72(6):413–4, 419–20.
3. Kennedy DW. Prognostic factors, outcomes, and staging in ethmoid sinus surgery. Laryngoscope 1992;102(12 Pt 2 Suppl 57):1–18.
4. Vleming M, de Vries N. Endoscopic paranasal sinus surgery: results. Am J Rhinol 1990;4:13–7.
5. Bernstein JM, Lebowitz RA, Jacobs JB. Initial report on postoperative healing after endoscopic sinus surgery with the microdebrider. Otolaryngol Head Neck Surg 1998;118(6):800–3.
6. Krouse JH, Christmas DA Jr. Powered instrumentation in functional endoscopic sinus surgery. II: a comparative study. Ear Nose Throat J 1996;75(1):42–4.
7. Hepworth EJ, Bucknor M, Patel A, et al. Nationwide survey on the use of image-guided functional endoscopic sinus surgery. Otolaryngol Head Neck Surg 2006; 135(1):68–73.
8. Orlandi RR. Image guidance: a survey of attitudes and use. Am J Rhinol 2006; 20(4):406–11.
9. Smith TL, Stewart MG, Orlandi RR, et al. Indications for image-guided sinus surgery: the current evidence. Am J Rhinol 2007;21(1):80–3.
10. Kaplan AV, Baim DS, Smith JJ, et al. Medical device development: from prototype to regulatory approval. Circulation 2004;109(25):3068–72.
11. Wang SS, Mendelson DN, Schulman KA, et al. Exploring options for improving healthcare. Am Heart J 2004;147(1):23–30.
12. Maisel WH. Medical device regulation: an introduction for the practicing physician. Ann Intern Med 2004;140(4):296–302.
13. Orlandi RR, Marple BF. Development and evaluation of new technologies in otolaryngology–head and neck surgery. Otolaryngol Head Neck Surg 2007; 137(4):529–31.
14. CPT process – How a code becomes a code. 2008. Available at: www.ama-assn. org/ama/pub/category/3882.html. Accessed September 24, 2006.
15. Casler JD. Clinical use of new technologies without scientific studies. Arch Otolaryngol Head Neck Surg 2003;129(6):674–7.
16. Gates GA. Surgical innovation and research. Arch Otolaryngol Head Neck Surg 2003;129(12):1352–3 [author reply 1354].

Evolution of the Endoscope and Endoscopic Sinus Surgery

Rakesh K. Chandra, MD*, David B. Conley, MD, Robert C. Kern, MD

KEYWORDS

- Sino-nasal endoscopy • Video technology
- Endoscopic sinus surgery • Hopkins rod • Digital imaging

HISTORICAL PERSPECTIVE

In 1879 Nitze is credited with the development of a small cystoscope[1] that was subsequently used by Hirschman in 1901 for visualization of the maxillary sinus via an oroantral fistula.[2] It had a small electric bulb and its use was mainly diagnostic. At approximately the same time, Reichert used a 7-mm endoscope in the surgical treatment of oroantral fistulas.[3] Visualization of the maxillary sinus with an antroscope via inferior meatal access was published by Spielberg in 1922.[4] Several years later in 1925, Maltz coined the term "sinuscopy" in promoting use of the endoscope for diagnosis.[5] These early endoscopes were severely limited in depth of field, optical quality, and low illumination from flame or small electric bulbs (**Fig. 1**). Many years later when the surgical microscope became available, Heermann published on the use of the microscopic for endonasal procedures in 1958.[6]

Substantial technologic improvements in fiberoptic design in the early 1950s enabled Harold H. Hopkins of Imperial College London to develop the rod optic endoscope, which became available in the early 1960s.[7] The Hopkins rod endoscopes greatly enhanced light delivery and optical quality. Further improvements came when Karl Storz from Tuttlingen, Germany, built endoscopes with angled views from 0° to 30°, 70°, 90°, and 120°.

These superior endoscopes with fiberoptic cold light and endoscopic cameras provided Messerklinger with the necessary tools to compile the major reference "Endoscopy of the nose," published in 1978.[8] The Messerklinger technique, which was only mentioned briefly in the book, shifted the focus of surgery from radical

Northwestern Sinus & Allergy Center, Department of Otolaryngology-Head & Neck Surgery, Northwestern University Feinberg School of Medicine, 675 North Street Clair, Galter 15-200, Chicago, IL 60611, USA
* Corresponding author.
E-mail address: rchandra@nmff.org (R.K. Chandra).

Otolaryngol Clin N Am 42 (2009) 747–752
doi:10.1016/j.otc.2009.07.010
0030-6665/09/$ – see front matter © 2009 Elsevier Inc. All rights reserved.

oto.theclinics.com

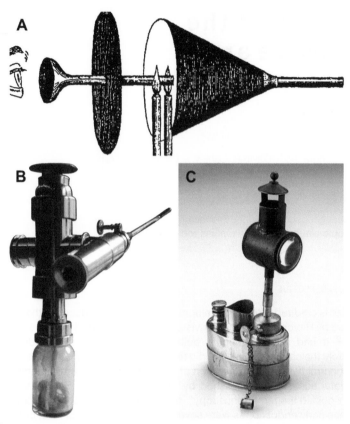

Fig. 1. (*A*) Principle of early endoscope and illumination source. (*Courtesy of* Karl Storz, Tuttlingen, Germany.) (*B*) Desormeaux endoscope (nineteenth century, London). (*Courtesy of* Karl Storz, Tuttlingen, Germany.) (*C*) Weiss light source (nineteenth century, London). (*Courtesy of* Karl Storz, private collection of Dr H.C. Mult, Sybill Storz, Tuttlingen, Germany.)

procedures of the dependent sinuses to focused treatment of the site of obstruction. Stammberger, Draf, Wigand, and others then adapted use of the endoscope to endonasal procedures, and Kennedy coined the term "functional endoscopic sinus surgery" in 1985.[9]

The historic effect of the introduction of the endoscope in endonasal sinus surgery is best put by Stammberger, "To put it bluntly, the endoscope emerged as the instrument that helped avoid unnecessary and unnecessarily radical surgery."[10]

MODERN ADVANCES

Advances in endoscopic technology have encompassed technologic innovations in all parts to the circuit, including light source, the telescope itself, camera head, camera processor, and monitor. Application of endoscopic technique has also proliferated in parallel with the technology to capture and archive photos and streaming video. In this section, the authors highlight key technical aspects of these advancements.

The quality of an endoscope image is determined first by the source data, the surgical field itself. Increased bleeding in the surgical field will oversaturate the image, diminishing quality. This digression is important to consider, however, because the use of a quality circuit may potentially avert maneuvers that confound surgical precision, thereby reducing intraoperative hemorrhage. The advent of the xenon light source (peak wavelengths in the 800–1000 nm range) has markedly augmented visualization simply by increasing the light output. This issue has been studied in automobile headlights, where brightness of xenon sources has been observed to be 3 times greater than that of standard halogen sources, with white rather than yellow tinted light quality. Compared with halogen light, xenon is more durable and efficient, with greater life, less heat production, and less energy consumption.

The Hopkins rod telescope is unique in that it employs true optical media (a series of glass rods and lenses) rather than fiberoptics. The advantage is a clear rather than pixilated image (**Fig. 1**A, B). In addition, autofocusing cameras tend to focus on the pixels rather than the target of interest, further diminishing image quality (**Fig. 1**C). The Hopkins rod telescope also affords greater illumination, color contrast, and depth perception. Current endoscopes have been manufactured at viewing angles ranging from 0° to 120°, with diameters at small as 2 mm. Other advances in the telescope itself have included offset angled endoscopes where the light cable attachment has been modified. Typically the light cable attachment is 180° from the direction to which the lens angle is biased. Manufacturing has allowed for repositioning of this attachment either 0° or 90° from the angle of view, thereby reducing the presence of the light cable in the surgeon's manual working field (**Fig. 2**A, B).

Enhancements of digital camera technology have paralleled those for camera technology in common applications. Digital cameras use chips that process color information. Earlier technology employed 1-chip cameras where all color information was processed together, resulting in significant limitations in contrast and balance. Modern 3-chip cameras have spate chips to process each of the 3 primary colors, red, blue, and green. This markedly enhances video quality, but this definition is often lost when video clips are saved and archived, secondary to postprocessing by digital compression algorithms.

Endoscopic surgery has also benefited from enhancements of the viewing monitor. This is of crucial importance because it is common practice for surgeons to use the monitor as the basis of visualization during surgery. Standard definition monitors have used a 4:3 aspect ratio, with pixel density of 640 × 480 in horizontal and vertical dimensions, respectively. In contrast, high-definition monitors use a 16:9 aspect ratio

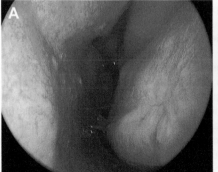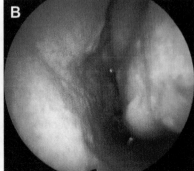

Fig. 2. (A) Left nasal cavity as seen using a 0° Hopkins rod telescope. (B) Same area observed by flexible fiberoptic endoscopy with an identical camera and light source. Note the diminished color definition and contrast. Focusing of the camera tends to highlight the fibers, creating graininess.

and 1920 × 1080 pixel density. This 7-fold enhancement significantly improves visualization of color and contrast definition, and the augmented aspect ratio improves peripheral visualization within the surgical field.

High-definition cameras also use a scheme of progressive scanning, rather than interlaced scanning, which maximizes image quality on the monitor display. Interlaced scanning is a traditional (analog) technology where each frame is scanned in 2 fields, each containing a series of 262 lines (one frame is the odd lines and the other frame is the even lines). In the United States, video stream is displayed at 60 Hz, or 60 fields per second (NTSC interlacing). Each pair of fields is superimposed through the interlaced scanning process, such that this translates to 30 frames per second. International television uses an interlacing scheme of 312 lines and 50 fields, or 25 frames per second (PAL interlacing). Interlaced scanning suffers from twitter (flickering) of the image, and attempts to compensate for this resulting in some blurring of the image quality and loss of detail. In contrast, progressive scanning reads and displays each line (row of pixels) sequentially, and updates the image at a rate of 60 frames per second. In comparison with 30 interlaced frames per second, this markedly improves image resolution, and lack of image flicker reduces the surgeon's visual fatigue. Another advantage of progressive scanning is that high-resolution still photographs can be captured for archiving.

The advantage of high-definition video has been demonstrated in an animal model of laparoscopic surgery, where 53 participants (mostly attending and fellow-level surgeons) subjectively graded high-definition camera/monitor systems as superior to standard definition with regard to anatomic orientation, instrument introduction, color, detail, and sharpness. A subset of this group (n = 20) also underwent skills assessment on a laparoscopic training simulator, including standardized tasks of hand-eye coordination, suturing, and knot tying. This analysis revealed significant performance advantage during knot tying with use of a high-definition camera/ monitor. This improvement was more pronounced in less experienced operators, underscoring the advantage of high-quality visualization modalities in accelerating the learning curve.[11]

NEW FRONTIERS

The basic set of diagnostic and operating endoscopes have changed little in the last 50 years. Small improvements have been made in optics and light-carrying capacity (**Fig. 3**A, B). The introduction of 45° scopes have fine tuned the angle necessary for frontal sinus work while reducing the optical distortion inherent in the 70° scopes that makes them so awkward to use.[12] These 45° scopes, with improved light-carrying capacity, and a wider angle of view provide the surgeon with the optimal instrument for most frontal sinus work.

One limitation in the conventional endoscope is the two-dimensional view obtained of the surgical anatomy. Despite much effort, numerous attempts at engineering binocular view or three-dimensional visualization via endoscopes for endoscopic sinus surgery have failed. Several techniques including dual channel endoscopes, shutters, dual cameras, and computer generated three-dimensional effects have not yet overcome the complex optical physics puzzle to provide a surgically useful image.[13] The need for angled views in sinus endoscopy only complicates the problem and combined with the surgical demands of a rotating field of visualization and anatomic limitations in the amount of space for instrumentation, this remains a substantial technical challenge. Nevertheless, research and development continue in this area including chip tip technology and high-definition video systems holding promise for useful results.

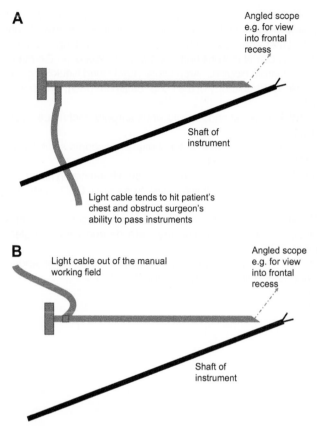

Fig. 3. (A) Conventional angled telescope where the cable attachment is 180° from the tip's bevel. (B) Offset telescopes afford the surgeon greater degrees of freedom in the surgical field during the introduction of instruments.

Another area of technological refinement in endoscopy is the development of very small fiber endoscopes. These scopes have fibers smaller than a millimeter and may allow visualization of paranasal sinuses either before surgical intervention or postoperatively when stenotic or small ostia limit conventional rigid or flexible endoscopes. These fibers have some flexibility, although they cannot presently tolerate highly angled bends. Although the optics are not likely to reach the refinement of the much larger commercially available flexible fiberoptic endoscopes, the ability to visualize the larger paranasal sinuses for diagnostic purposes without surgical intervention is intriguing.

REFERENCES

1. Woodham J. History of the development of surgery for sinusitis. In: Donald PJ, Gluckman JL, Rice DH, editors. The sinuses. New York: Raven; 1995. p. 3–14.
2. Hirschmann A. Über Endoskopie der Nase und deren Nebenhöhlen. Eine neue Untersuchungsmethode. Arch Laryngol Rhinol (Berl) 1903;14:195–7 [in German].
3. Reichert M. Über eine neue Unterscuhungsmethode der Oberkieferhöhle mittels des Antroskops. Berl klin Wochenschr 1902;401:478 [in German].

4. Spielberg W. Antroscopy of the maxillary sinus. Laryngoscope 1922;32:441–4.
5. Maltz M. New instrument: the sinuscope. Laryngoscope 1925;35:805–11.
6. Heerman H. Uber endonasale chirurgie unter verwendung des binocularen mikroskopes. Arch Ohr Nas Kehlkopfheilk 1958;171:295–7 [in German].
7. Jennings CR. Harold Hopkins. Arch Otolaryngol Head Neck Surg 1998;124:1042.
8. Messerklinger W. Endoscopy of the nose. Baltimore (MD): Urban and Schwarzenberg; 1978.
9. Kennedy DW. Functional endoscopic sinus surgery: technique. Arch Otolaryngol 1985;111:643–9.
10. Stammberger H. The evolution of functional endoscopic sinus surgery. Ear Nose Throat J 1994;73(7):451, 454–5.
11. Hagiike M, Phillips EH, Berci G. Performance differences in laparoscopic surgical skills between true high-definition and three-chip CCD video systems. Surg Endosc 2007;21:1849–54.
12. Kang SK, White PS, Lee MS, et al. A randomized control trial of surgical task performance in frontal recess surgery: zero degree versus angled telescopes. Am J Rhinol 2002;16(1):33–6.
13. Kennedy DW. Technical innovations and the evolution of endoscopic sinus surgery. Ann Otol Rhinol Laryngol Suppl 2006;196:3–12.

Imaging of the Paranasal Sinuses and In-Office CT

Paul D. Campbell, Jr, MD, S. James Zinreich, MD*, Nafi Aygun, MD

KEYWORDS

- Imaging for FESS • Sinus anatomy • Sinusitis
- Cone beam CT • CT dose-Index

Since the introduction of functional endoscopic sinus surgery (FESS) in the United States in 1985, the information gained from imaging of the nasal cavity and paranasal sinuses has proved imperative in understanding the regional morphology and guidance of surgical procedures. This regional morphology can vary significantly from patient to patient, and one quickly becomes aware of the fact that "no two noses are alike."

Given the need for accurate and detailed display of the nasal cavity and paranasal sinus anatomy, the commonly used imaging technology in 1985, standard plain films and polytomography, was quickly replaced with CT. Coronal CT scans afforded improved resolution of the bony framework and the superimposed mucosa in addition to regional inflammatory pathology. The application of multiplanar reconstruction and then 3-D imaging subsequently provided a more 3-D understanding of the CT imaging data.

In 1991 a significant advance in the use of imaging information to help guide surgeons in the performance of FESS was accomplished with the introduction of image-guided surgery. The imaging data were used to register a patient's location on the operating table with the patient's imaging data in a computer, which then was able to show the location of the surgeon's instruments in the operating field. Surgical accuracy and safety were significantly advanced.

More than 20 years after the introduction of FESS in the United States, the importance of imaging for surgeons continues to be the anatomic detail afforded by this technology, the roadmap it provides in planning the surgery, and the morphologic detail it provides in patients with recurrent disease after surgery. When considering the need to distinguish between various pathologic entities, MRI information can be added to CT information, because its soft tissue resolution is superior to CT.

The Russell H. Morgan Department of Radiology and Radiological Sciences, The Johns Hopkins Medical Institutions, 600 North Wolfe Street/Phipps B-112, Baltimore, MD 21287, USA
* Corresponding author.
E-mail address: sjzinreich@jhmi.edu (S.J. Zinreich).

Otolaryngol Clin N Am 42 (2009) 753–764
doi:10.1016/j.otc.2009.08.015
0030-6665/09/$ – see front matter © 2009 Published by Elsevier Inc.

oto.theclinics.com

The latest development in CT technology is cone beam CT (CBCT) instrumentation.[1] This is a miniaturized CT scanner providing sufficient resolution to outline the maxillofacial bony architecture, and therefore the nasal cavity and paranasal sinus morphology. This scanner requires little space, is easy to operate, emits reduced radiation, and can easily fit in an office setting. This equipment may change the way imaging of the nasal cavity and paranasal sinuses will be performed in the future. These developments are the topics discussed in this article.

CT TECHNIQUE

Single-channel CT scanners use incremental or helical acquisition schemes for paranasal sinus examinations. Image acquisition in the coronal plane is preferred for optimal display of the anterior osteomeatal unit. The slice thickness should be 3 mm or less without interslice gap for optimal evaluation. Image acquisition in the coronal plane may require extension of the head, which may not be possible for some elderly patients and patients with airway problems or neck pain. Thin axial images can be reconstructed in the coronal plane for such patients.

Multidetector CT (MDCT) scanners (also called multichannel or multislice CT scanners) use multiple rows of detectors that allow registration of multiple channels of data with one rotation of the x-ray tube. For example, a 16-slice MDCT scanner has a 16-fold capacity for collecting image data per x-ray tube rotation compared with a single-channel CT. Currently, 64-channel CT scanners are in routine clinical use. A head-to-toe CT scan with slices as thin as 0.2 mm can be obtained in 60 seconds. Recently, 312-channel scanners have been introduced that can image the same volume of tissue over and over again in a short time affording the physiologic studies of heart motion, myocardial perfusion, and brain perfusion. Thin slices permit isotropic data sets, in which the voxels (the smallest elements of a data set) are cubical. Isotropic voxels afford excellent reconstruction of images in essentially any desired plane without degradation of image quality. Isotropic imaging created a paradigm shift in CT imaging, no longer limited by the plane of acquisition. Data can be collected from a body part in any desired plane and 2-D images in any desired plane (multiplanar reconstruction) can be reconstructed (**Fig. 1**). Real-time interactive manipulation of image data and 3-D reconstructions are made possible by high-performance workstations equipped with special software.

In the MDCT scanners, the x-ray beam is collimated to the thickness of the detector row making it a fan-shaped beam.

Flat panel–based/CBCT scanners were recently introduced for routine clinical use. Instead of rows of detectors, these use detectors arranged in a flat surface to capture the x-ray, which is not collimated to a fan shape but rather takes the form of a cone. These scanners have changed the image acquisition paradigm once again. Flat panel–based CT, instead of building the volume from individual slices, acquires the image data volume directly. This provides seamless volume images, which improve 2-D and 3-D reconstructions and model-building capability for presurgical evaluation.

The x-ray source and the detector rotate around a fixed region of interest. The flat panel area detector permits a wider Z-axis coverage compared with a CT slice, allowing coverage of large areas in just one turn of the gantry, with enough data acquired to permit image reconstruction. A CBCT system (**Fig. 2**) has some advantages over traditional MDCT, including decreased cost and radiation exposure. It also has inherent disadvantages, however, which include poor soft tissue contrast resolution due to noise from scatter radiation. Modern MDCT scanners have a contrast resolution of 1 Hounsfield unit (HU), which is 10 times better than that afforded by CBCT scanners. This remains the most significant barrier in widespread clinical use of CBCT.

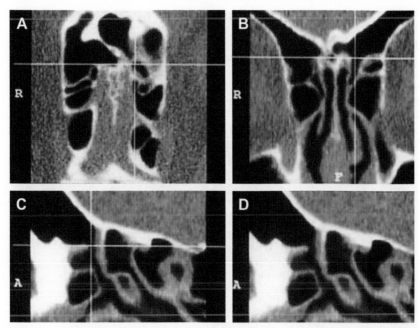

Fig. 1. Multiplanar reconstruction of isotropic imaging data in the axial (*A*), coronal (*B*), and sagittal (*C, D*) planes reveals high-resolution reconstructed imaging information whereby the reconstructed planes are indistinguishable from the acquisition plane. The cross hairs (*A–C*) reveal the ease of cross-referencing anatomic information.

In-office Considerations

The implementation of this technology in a rhinologic office would be more convenient for patients requiring the study, in that it would preclude the need to go through the effort of an additional office appointment. Although the immediate availability of the imaging data improves physician convenience, there are additional factors that need to be considered before adding this equipment to an ear, nose, and throat (ENT) office. The financial considerations regarding the equipment purchase are beyond the scope of this article, which addresses only technical issues.

Before a practice considers acquiring CBCT technology, perhaps the first issue to be considered is whether or not a facility is capable of housing the equipment. As CBCT emits radiation, there are radiation safety considerations, which must be evaluated on a state-by-state basis, as laws vary. Radiation monitoring is important to minimize exposure to the office staff and the general public, requiring proper structural shielding of the equipment to limit the scatter radiation beyond the space housing the equipment.

Most scanners permit the manipulation and viewing of the acquired data at the workstation, but if there is a desire to view images at other locations, a high-speed network must be in place. The amount of data acquired is often large and, depending on the volume of the practice, considerations must be made in regard to data storage. Accessibility of the images from multiple locations, such as office, operating room, and so forth, requires the use of a picture archiving and communications system and compatibility of this equipment with existing equipment should be considered.

It is also important to consider who will actually be acquiring the images. In most cases, a licensed CT technologist is needed to operate the equipment. Furthermore,

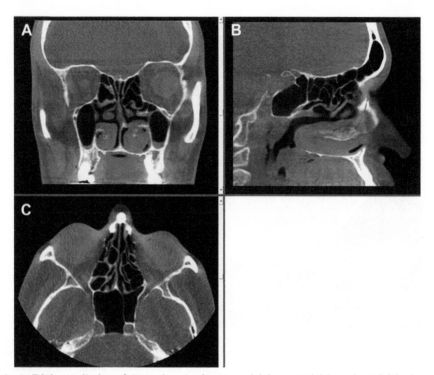

Fig. 2. Triplanar display of CBCT data in the coronal (*A*), sagittal (*B*), and axial (*C*) planes demonstrating good resolution of the bony morphology of the nasal cavity and paranasal sinuses.

who will interpret the imaging information? Although dental specialists may be well trained in the interpretation of the dental applications and otolaryngologists in sinus applications, what about nondental and nonsinus lesions that occasionally are present? The lack of soft tissue contrast, hence the inability to diagnose soft tissue lesions in the paranasal sinuses and orbits, is a significant limitation that has the potential to increase the vulnerability of practitioners. Liability issues regarding "missed" diagnoses need to be considered and need to be addressed in the implementation process of this diagnostic equipment. Lastly, but of equal importance, is the consideration of the frequency of use of the equipment. Having the equipment on the premises of an office makes it convenient to evaluate patients with chronic sinusitis with this technology. The physician-owner of the equipment needs to address possible queries regarding "overutilization" and "self-referral." Strict guidelines regarding this issue should be established at the time of implementation of this technology to show a planned approach to the CT usage and therefore avoid possible criticisms that may be raised.

Radiation Considerations

To measure radiation emitted by MDCT scanners in a standardized fashion, CT dose-index (CTDI) and dose-length product have been developed. Approximate radiation equivalent doses related to diagnostic procedures are provided in **Table 1**.[2] The same general radiation principles are considered when comparing CBCT to MDCT but conventional metrics, such as CTDI and dose-length product, cannot be directly

Table 1
Radiation dose comparison

Diagnostic Procedure	Effective Dose (mSv)	Number of Equivalent Posteroanterior Chest Radiographs for Equivalent Dose	Time Period for Equivalent Effective Dose from Natural Background Radiation
Posterioanterior chest radiograph	0.02	1	2.4 days
Skull radiograph	0.07	4	8.5 days
Lumbar spine	1.30	65	158 days
Intravenous pyelogram	2.50	125	304 days
Upper gastrointestinal series	3.00	150	1.0 year
Barium enema	7.00	350	2.3 years
CT head/sinuses	2.00/0.96	100/48	243/100 + days
CT abdomen	10.00	500	3.3 years

Data from FDA. Available at: www.fda.gov/cdrh/ct/risks.html.

applied to CBCT because of altered beam geometry and differences in x-ray scatter profiles. In addition, the standard phantoms used do not capture the expanded Z-axis beam generated by CBCT that potentially results in significant underestimation of the dose associated with CBCT. An additional complicating factor is that the highest radiation dose in CBCT is at the center of the field, with diminished radiation toward the periphery. For these reasons, volumetric CTDI and dose-length product have been introduced to estimate radiation exposure with CBCT but as yet there is no universally applicable and standardized measure available. Nonetheless, actual dose measurements are obtained with volumetric indices using 18-cm phantoms with a few additional centimeters to incorporate scatter radiation that inevitably are encountered. Comparisons between CBCT and traditional MDCT have been performed (**Table 2**). To maintain the same signal to noise at thinner slice sections, more radiation dose must be used. Published reports indicate that the effective dose varies for various full field-of-view (FOV) CBCT devices, ranging from 0.29 to 0.477 mSv, depending on the type and model of CBCT equipment, the duration of exposure, and FOV selected (see **Table 2**). Comparing these doses with multiples of a single panoramic dose or background equivalent radiation dose, CBCT provides an equivalent patient radiation dose of 5 to 74 times that of a single film–based panoramic x ray or 3 to 48 days of background radiation. The use of additional personal protection (thyroid collar) can substantially reduce the dose by up to 40%.

Table 2
Cone beam CT effective doses for paranasal sinus procedures

Current (mA)	Duration of Exposure (Seconds)	Effective Dose (mSv)
1	7.8	0.03
3.8	7.8	0.10
3.8	20	0.20
3.8	40	0.55

Comparison with patient dose reported for maxillofacial/sinus imaging by MDCT, approximately 1.0 mSv, indicates that CBCT provides a dose reduction. It is not yet clear, however, whether or not the reported degree of dose reduction will be realized in routine clinical settings.

APPLICATIONS OF CONE BEAM CT

Given the ease with which it evaluates the maxillofacial area and its bony resolution, CBCT is used in the assessment of bony and dental pathologic conditions, including fracture, structural maxillofacial deformity, preoperative assessment of impacted teeth, and the temporomandibular joints.[3] It is also used to evaluate availability of bone for implant placement. The technology can also be used to assist in the computer-aided design and manufacture of implant prosthetics,[4] although less than perfect results have been reported with model-forming capability.[5]

It is only natural to expect that CBCT-generated images can be used for surgical navigation during endoscopic sinus surgery. The accuracy of the existing intraoperative stereotactic guidance systems using CBCT images has not been thoroughly investigated; however, some preliminary work suggests feasibility in this regard.[6] The limited FOV and inability to include all fiducial markers seem to be the main practical barrier in front of CBCT's use for all sinus procedures. Regarding endoscopic sinus and skull base surgery, there has been an increasing need for efficient intraoperative real-time imaging, which would show the anatomic changes resulting from surgery. A C-arm–mounted CBCT affords a means to address this need. It provides excellent morphologic localization with high spatial orientation of vital structures during surgery with a potential to increase surgical precision and decrease surgical complications and the need for a repeated surgical procedure, which would otherwise be unforeseen without the use of this instrumentation.[7–10]

MRI TECHNIQUE

The most significant advantage of MRI over CT is its superior contrast resolution, which allows differentiation of sinus inflammatory disease from mass lesions, brain, and orbital structures. Evaluation of neoplastic and invasive inflammatory processes of the paranasal sinuses is best accomplished by MRI. MRI, however, often fails to evaluate the integrity of the bony architecture precluding its use as a roadmap to guide FESS.

T1- and T2-weighted MRI obtained in axial and coronal planes provide a satisfactory evaluation of the sinuses and their mucosa. Contrast-enhanced (gadolinium-diethylenetriamine pentaacetic acid), fat-saturated, T1-weighted images are indispensable for a more comprehensive examination, especially in patients with noninflammatory sinus pathology.

ANATOMY

An understanding of the physiology of the nasal cycle and the mucocilliary clearance of the respective paranasal sinuses is a requisite for understanding the osteomeatal chanels, which provide an intercommunication between the nasal cavity and the paranasal sinuses. The anatomic evaluation needs to focus on the three tight spots: the frontal recess, the infundibulum–middle meatus, and the sphenoethmoid recess.

The frontal sinus drainage pathway is the most complex. The bottom portion of the hourglass-shaped frontal sinus drainage pathway is the frontal recess and also one of the narrowest channels of this outflow tract (the first tight spot) **(Fig. 3)**. The structures

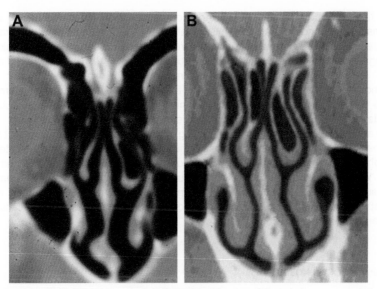

Fig. 3. Coronal CT image in the plane of the frontal recess (*A*) and the corresponding 3-D image (*B*), demonstrating the most anterior tight spot.

adjacent to the frontal recess are the agger nasi cell anteriorly, the ethmoid bulla posteriorly, and the uncinate process inferiorly. The agger nasi cell is an ethmoturbinal remnant, which is present in almost all patients. It is aerated and represents the most anterior ethmoid air cell. It, and frontal cells, usually border the frontal recess; thus, its size may directly influence the patency of the frontal recess and the anterior middle meatus. Anteriorly, the uncinate process fuses with the posteromedial wall of the agger nasi cell and the posteromedial wall of the nasolacrimal duct. Laterally, the free edge of the uncinate process delimits the infundibulum, which is the air passage that connects the maxillary sinus ostium to the middle meatus (the second tight spot).

The superior attachment of the uncinate process has three major variations that determine the anatomic configuration of the frontal recess and its drainage.[11] These variations are

- The uncinate process may extend laterally to attach to the lamina papyracea or the ethmoid bulla, forming a terminal recess of the infundibulum; the frontal recess opens directly to the middle meatus (recessus terminalis).
- The uncinate process may extend medially and attach to the lateral surface of the middle turbinate.
- The uncinate process may extend medially and superiorly to attach directly to the skull base.

In the latter two forms, the frontal recess drains to the infundibulum (recessus frontalis).

The sphenoethmoidal recess (the third tight spot) receives drainage from the posterior ethmoid cells and the sphenoid sinus. It lies just lateral to the nasal septum and leads to the posterior aspect of the superior meatus. The sphenoethmoidal recess is visualized on coronal images but is best evaluated in the sagittal and axial planes.

Using a coronal CT scan, the anatomy of the frontal recess, infundibulum, and middle meatus can be visualized. This is crucial for proper diagnosis and treatment.

Using the real-time multiplanar reconstruction capabilities of modern imaging workstations, understanding of the complex anatomy of these regions can be advanced considerably. The authors found oblique coronal reconstructions with 20° craniocaudal angulation and oblique sagittal reconstructions with 5° to 10° lateromedial angulation particularly helpful in demonstrating the frontal-recess–agger nasi cell–uncinate process relationship. Routine axial images show the sphenoethmoidal recess to the authors' satisfaction but minimally obliqued sagittal reconstructions best demonstrate the sphenoethmoidal recess–superior meatus relationship.

The authors prefer to evaluate the imaging information starting with the most anterior images showing the frontal sinuses and systematically proceeding posteriorly through the sphenoid sinus specifically studying the anatomy surrounding the tight spots. With completion of this task, an evaluation focusing on the nasal septum and proceeding laterally affords additional information regarding the osteomeatal channels, specifically the turbinate relationship to the uncinate process, frontal cells, and anterior and posterior ethmoid cells.[12,13]

APPEARANCE OF RHINOSINUSITIS

The most common indication for sinus imaging is chronic rhinosinusitis (CRS). CT is the imaging standard for evaluation of CRS.[14] The CT signs suggestive of CRS include diffuse or focal mucosal thickening, with partial or complete opacification of the paranasal sinuses; bone remodeling with uniform thickening caused by osteitis from adjacent chronic mucosal inflammation; and polyposis. Thickening and sclerosis of the bony walls of the sinuses are at least in part secondary to the spread of the inflammation through the haversian system within the bone.[15,16]

The distribution of the inflammatory mucosal changes in the nasal cavity and sinuses may provide a clue to the focus of mechanical obstruction, which can be pinpointed by evaluating the sinus drainage pathways. Although CT provides excellent information about the extent and distribution of mucosal disease and the status of the nasal air passages, it does not yield much information regarding the cause of the changes (eg, infection, allergies, granulomatous inflammation, postsurgical scarring, and so forth).

In the acute state, the viscosity of the inflammatory process is of intermediate attenuation on CT (10–25 HU). In the more chronic state, sinus secretions become thickened and concentrated, and the CT attenuation increases, with density measurements of 30 to 60 HU.[17] In the acute state, the obstruction of a specific sinus is followed by a circumferential mucosal edema/inflammation and fluid exudation, represented on CT by an air fluid level and uniform circumferential soft tissue thickening. Contrasted CT and T1-weighted MRI show a uniform uninterrupted enhancement adjacent to the peripheral sinus bony outline. This is characteristic of an inflammatory process within the paranasal sinuses.

Antrochoanal and sphenochoanal polyps appear as well-defined masses that arise from the maxillary or sphenoid sinus and extend to the choana through the middle meatus or sphenoethmoid recess, respectively. They can present as nasopharyngeal masses. It is important to recognize their origin and relationship to the maxillary or sphenoid ostium in treatment planning.

Retention cysts are common incidental findings on imaging studies and are seen as well-defined rounded masses, typically on the maxillary sinus floor. Their clinical significance is not clear.[18] They may become symptomatic if large enough to interfere with drainage pathways.[19]

Mucocele, a complication of CRS, results from a persistant obstruction of the sinus drainage and subsequent expansion of the sinus. Mucoceles are seen more commonly in the ethmoid and frontal sinuses and present with symptoms secondary to compression of the adjacent structures, in addition to the usual symptoms of CRS.

On MRI the appearance of AFS is due to the concentration of feromagnetic elements as described by Zinreich and colleagues,[20] and demonstrated in **Fig. 4**. Som and Curtin[17] describe four patterns of MRI signal intensity that can be seen with chronic sinusitis:

- Hypointense on T1-weighted images and hyperintense on T2-weighted images with a protein concentration of less than 9%
- Hyperintense on T1-weighted images and hyperintense on T2-weighted images with total protein concentration increased to 20% to 25%
- Hyperintense on T1-weighted images and hypointense on T2-weighted images with total protein concentration of 25% to 30%
- Hypointense on T1-weighted images and T2-weighted images with a protein concentration greater than 30% and inspissated secretions in an almost solid form

MRI of inspissated secretions (ie, those with protein concentrations greater than 30%) may have a pitfall in that the signal voids on T1- and T2-weighted images may look identical to normally aerated sinuses.

The correlation between patient symptoms and CT findings is difficult to determine partly because chronic mucosal inflammation may be present without CT findings and asymptomatic persons can have abnormal CT scans. Several studies failed to show a correlation between symptom severity and severity of CT findings.[21–25] In particular, symptoms, such as headache and facial pain, do not correlate with CT findings at all.[26,27] A positive correlation between the severity of symptoms and CT findings may be demonstrated when certain symptoms and negative CT examinations are eliminated.[28,29] The nasal endoscopy findings correlate with CT findings, although the correlation is less than perfect.[24,30,31] The positive predictive value of abnormal endoscopy for abnormal CT is greater than 90%, whereas the negative predictive value of normal endoscopy for normal CT is only 70%.[24,26]

The impact of CT on treatment decision was evaluated in a small study.[32] CT changed the treatment in one third of the patients and allowed more agreement on treatment plan among ENT surgeons.[32]

NEOPLASMS OF THE SINONASAL CAVITIES

Squamous cell carcinoma arising from the sinonasal epithelium accounts for 80% of the malignant tumors seen in this area. Adenocarcinomas arising from the minor

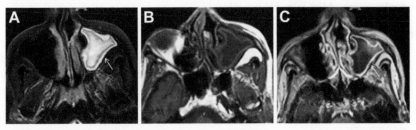

Fig. 4. T2-weighted image (*A*), T1-weighted image (*B*), and postcontrast T1-weighted image. (*C*) These images reveal the typical acute inflammatory change with sinus contents showing fluid-like signal and enhancing mucosa (*arrow*).

salivary glands interspersed in the sinonasal mucosa account for up to 10% of the malignant tumors. Melanomas are responsible for 5% of sinonasal malignant tumors. Less common malignant tumors of the sinonasal cavities include olfactory neuroblastoma, lymphomas, and sarcomas. A detailed discussion of these individual entities is beyond the scope of this article.

On CT, neoplasms are recognized by their invasive character and bone erosion. Focal bone erosion with or without expansion is evident. Depending on size and extension, the mass may erode through the bony confines of a particular sinus and invade the tissues peripheral to the sinus bony architecture. The precise extension can be best determined with a contrast-enhanced MRI study. The mass is usually of lower signal intensity and its contrast enhancement is less than that of an inflammatory process. The uniform enhancement seen peripherally within a sinus cavity with inflammation is interrupted as the mass extends beyond the confines of the sinus cavity. Additionally, certain characteristics are associated with specific neoplasms. Peripheral cysts are associated with esthesioneuroblastomas. A serpiginous cerebral sulcal–like enhancement is associated with inverted papilomas.

SUMMARY

Two and a half decades after the introduction of FESS in the United States, the role of imaging with respect to this surgical procedure is the information it provides regarding the anatomic detail of the nasal cavity and paranasal sinuses. The imaging information affords surgical planning and guidance. Furthermore, when considering the application of CT and MRI, the information derived from these technologies helps narrow the differential diagnosis and helps define the causes of various pathologic entities confronted in this area.

As FESS has evolved since 1985, so has imaging technology and its application with regards to this surgery. Of significant note is the introduction of image-guided surgery. Image guidance further revolutionized the use of imaging information in that it provided a direct confirmation of anatomic structures and improved the guidance and safety of the surgical act.

The introduction of CBCT begins a new phase of change in the use of imaging for the evaluation of maxillofacial pathology. Its presence in the office environment addresses issues related to the patient and physician "convenience factor." The radiation exposure and diagnostic issues are new topics with which ENT offices need to deal (in most instances for the first time), to adhere to the various regulatory measures and potential risks introduced by this technology in the in-office setting.

Regarding the use of CBCT in the OR setting, early results seem to show augmented benefits provided by image-guided surgery, in that it provides confirmation of the extent of surgery before patients leave the operating room, therefore providing accurate confirmation of the surgical objective.

REFERENCES

1. Mozzo P, Procacci C, Tacconi A, et al. A new volumetric CT machine for dental imaging based on the cone-beam technique: preliminary results. Eur Radiol 1998;8:1558–64.
2. FDA. Available at: www.fda.gov/cdrh/ct/risks.html.
3. Thomas SL. Application of cone-beam CT in the office setting. Dent Clin North Am 2008;52:753–9, vi.
4. Scarfe WC, Farman AG. What is cone-beam CT and how does it work? Dent Clin North Am 2008;52:707–30, v.

5. Hassan B, van der Stelt P, Sanderink G. Accuracy of three-dimensional measurements obtained from cone beam computed tomography surface-rendered images for cephalometric analysis: influence of patient scanning position. Eur J Orthod 2009;31:129–34.
6. Eggers G, Muhling J, Hofele C. Clinical use of navigation based on cone-beam computer tomography in maxillofacial surgery. Br J Oral Maxillofac Surg 2009.
7. Chan Y, Siewerdsen JH, Rafferty MA, et al. Cone-beam computed tomography on a mobile C-arm: novel intraoperative imaging technology for guidance of head and neck surgery. J Otolaryngol Head Neck Surg 2008;37:81–90.
8. Bachar G, Barker E, Nithiananthan S, et al. Three-dimensional tomosynthesis and cone-beam computed tomography: an experimental study for fast, low-dose intraoperative imaging technology for guidance of sinus and skull base surgery. Laryngoscope 2009;119:434–41.
9. Rafferty MA, Siewerdsen JH, Chan Y, et al. Intraoperative cone-beam CT for guidance of temporal bone surgery. Otolaryngol Head Neck Surg 2006;134:801–8.
10. Rafferty MA, Siewerdsen JH, Chan Y, et al. Investigation of C-arm cone-beam CT-guided surgery of the frontal recess. Laryngoscope 2005;115:2138–43.
11. Daniels DL, Mafee MF, Smith MM, et al. The frontal sinus drainage pathway and related structures. AJNR Am J Neuroradiol 2003;24:1618–27.
12. Zammit-Maempel I, Chadwick CL, Willis SP. Radiation dose to the lens of eye and thyroid gland in paranasal sinus multislice CT. Br J Radiol 2003;76:418–20.
13. Tack D, Widelec J, De Maertelaer V, et al. Comparison between low-dose and standard-dose multidetector CT in patients with suspected chronic sinusitis. AJR Am J Roentgenol 2003;181:939–44.
14. Benninger MS, Ferguson BJ, Hadley JA, et al. Adult chronic rhinosinusitis: definitions, diagnosis, epidemiology, and pathophysiology. Otolaryngol Head Neck Surg 2003;129:S1–32.
15. Perloff JR, Gannon FH, Bolger WE, et al. Bone involvement in sinusitis: an apparent pathway for the spread of disease. Laryngoscope 2000;110:2095–9.
16. Khalid AN, Hunt J, Perloff JR, et al. The role of bone in chronic rhinosinusitis. Laryngoscope 2002;112:1951–7.
17. Som PM, Curtin HD. Chronic inflammatory sinonasal diseases including fungal infections. The role of imaging. Radiol Clin North Am 1993;31:33–44.
18. Bhattacharyya N. Do maxillary sinus retention cysts reflect obstructive sinus phenomena? Arch Otolaryngol Head Neck Surg 2000;126:1369–71.
19. Hadar T, Shvero J, Nageris BI, et al. Mucus retention cyst of the maxillary sinus: the endoscopic approach. Br J Oral Maxillofac Surg 2000;38:227–9.
20. Zinreich S, Kennedy D, Malat J, et al. Diagnosis with CT and MR imaging. Radiology 1998;169(2):439–44.
21. Bhattacharyya T, Piccirillo J, Wippold FJ 2nd. Relationship between patient-based descriptions of sinusitis and paranasal sinus computed tomographic findings. Arch Otolaryngol Head Neck Surg 1997;123:1189–92.
22. Ashraf N, Bhattacharyya N. Determination of the "incidental" Lund score for the staging of chronic rhinosinusitis. Otolaryngol Head Neck Surg 2001;125:483–6.
23. Stewart MG, Sicard MW, Piccirillo JF, et al. Severity staging in chronic sinusitis: are CT scan findings related to patient symptoms? Am J Rhinol 1999;13:161–7.
24. Stankiewicz JA, Chow JM. Nasal endoscopy and the definition and diagnosis of chronic rhinosinusitis. Otolaryngol Head Neck Surg 2002;126:623–7.
25. Stankiewicz JA, Chow JM. A diagnostic dilemma for chronic rhinosinusitis: definition accuracy and validity. Am J Rhinol 2002;16:199–202.

26. Rosbe KW, Jones KR. Usefulness of patient symptoms and nasal endoscopy in the diagnosis of chronic sinusitis. Am J Rhinol 1998;12:167–71.

27. Mudgil SP, Wise SW, Hopper KD, et al. Correlation between presumed sinusitis-induced pain and paranasal sinus computed tomographic findings. Ann Allergy Asthma Immunol 2002;88:223–6.

28. Arango P, Kountakis SE. Significance of computed tomography pathology in chronic rhinosinusitis. Laryngoscope 2001;111:1779–82.

29. Kenny TJ, Duncavage J, Bracikowski J, et al. Prospective analysis of sinus symptoms and correlation with paranasal computed tomography scan. Otolaryngol Head Neck Surg 2001;125:40–3.

30. Rose GE, Sandy C, Hallberg L, et al. Clinical and radiologic characteristics of the imploding antrum, or "silent sinus," syndrome. Ophthalmology 2003;110:811–8.

31. Kennedy DW, Wright ED, Goldberg AN. Objective and subjective outcomes in surgery for chronic sinusitis. Laryngoscope 2000;110:29–31.

32. Anzai Y, Yueh B. Imaging evaluation of sinusitis: diagnostic performance and impact on health outcome. Neuroimaging Clin N Am 2003;13:251–63, xi.

Intraoperative Imaging for Otorhinolaryngology— Head and Neck Surgery

Seth Isaacs, MD, Samer Fakhri, MD, Amber Luong, MD, PhD,
Martin J. Citardi, MD*

KEYWORDS

- Image-guided surgery • Endoscopic sinus surgery
- Intraoperative imaging • Endoscopic skull base surgery
- Volume CT

Advances in endoscopic surgery have revolutionized the evaluation and management of sinonasal diseases over the last 2 decades. Experience with endoscopy has led to the application of endoscopic techniques to regions beyond the paranasal sinuses, including adjacent areas of the skull base. Endoscopic skull base surgical techniques, compared with traditional craniofacial approaches, may allow pathology in these regions to be treated with reduced morbidity. Technological advancements have preceded major improvements in paranasal sinus skull base surgery. The cornerstone of these technological improvements has been the rod-lens endoscope, which has enabled adequate visualization, illumination, and magnification within the paranasal sinuses as well as at the boundary of the paranasal sinuses at the anterior and middle skull base and orbit. Unfortunately, the rigid endoscopes only provide a two-dimensional (2D) representation of a complex three-dimensional (3D) space. Over the past 10 to 15 years, image-guided surgery has emerged as an important tool that compensates for at least some of the intrinsic limitations of surgical endoscopy. An important limitation of image-guided surgery is its dependence on a preoperative image data set. Obviously anatomic manipulation resulting from the surgical procedure is not represented in the preoperative imaging. Intraoperative imaging provides an opportunity to obtain near real-time information that can be used to update the navigation system data set and alter surgical decision-making. Advances in intraoperative imaging technology potentially may enhance the effectiveness and reduce the morbidity of endoscopic procedures of the paranasal sinuses and skull base.

Disclosures: Dr Citardi and Dr Fakhri are consultants for Medtronic ENT (Jacksonville, Florida).
Department of Otorhinolaryngology-Head and Neck Surgery, University of Texas Medical School at Houston, Texas Sinus Institute, Texas Skull Base Institute, 6431 Fannin Street, MSB 5.036, Houston, TX 77030, USA
* Corresponding author.
E-mail address: martin.j.citardi@uth.tmc.edu (M.J. Citardi).

Intraoperative imaging with or without image-guided surgery also has applications beyond standard endoscopic sinus surgery. By giving a real-time update for image-guided surgery, intraoperative imaging may permit even more extensive procedures of the skull base. Furthermore, intraoperative imaging may serve important roles in craniomaxillofacial procedures, including a role in reducing complex facial fractures. In this role, intraoperative imaging gives immediate information intraoperatively about the positioning of bony fragments and thus guides the surgeon for their optimal placement and fixation.

TERMINOLOGY

Nearly 20 years ago, the International Society for Computer Aided Surgery proposed a broad definition of computer-aided surgery:

The scope of Computer-Aided Surgery encompasses all fields within surgery, as well as biomedical imaging and instrumentation, and digital technology employed as an adjunct to imaging in diagnosis, therapeutics, and surgery. Topics featured include frameless as well as conventional stereotaxic procedures, surgery guided by ultrasound, image-guided focal irradiation, robotic surgery, and other therapeutic interventions that are performed with the use of digital imaging technology.[1]

Broadly speaking, computer-aided surgery encompasses all semiconductor-based technologies with surgical applications. Thus, computer-aided surgery includes surgical navigation, computer-aided image review, stereotactic surgery, robotic surgery, telemedicine, and electronic medical records.

Over the years, the term *image-guided surgery* has emerged as the preferred term for surgical navigation applications in endoscopic sinus surgery. From a practical standpoint, image-guided surgery includes both software-enabled review of imaging data as well as surgical navigation, since modern image-guided surgery systems easily support both applications during surgical procedures.

By default, diagnostic imaging, even if it is acquired using semiconductor-based technology, is not part of computer-aided surgery because, unlike computer-aided surgery, diagnostic imaging does not enable the surgeon to manipulate imaging data so as to develop a functional representation of the relative anatomy. Treating a computer like a digital light box for reviewing a CT scan is not computer-aided surgery; however, studying those images using various software tools, which may enable image reconstruction/segmentation and window level/width adjustments, is computer-aided surgery.

Intraoperative imaging refers to the acquisition of imaging data during actual surgical procedures. Because intraoperative imaging data is reviewed interactively at a computer workstation and then commonly uploaded for image-guided surgery, intraoperative imaging is part of computer-aided surgery.

EQUIPMENT FOR INTRAOPERATIVE IMAGING

Intraoperative imaging requires equipment for image acquisition and transfer as well as review and manipulation. In some scenarios, image-guided surgery will also be employed and, thus, the images from intraoperative imaging must be transferred to the image-guided surgery computer as well. A computer workstation is required to view and manipulate the intraoperative images; similar hardware is also a part of the image-acquisition process. Finally, software is needed to upload the newly acquired images into the navigation system.

The ideal requirements for intraoperative imaging include portability, rapid image acquisition, compatibility with commercially available image-guided surgery systems, and patient safety. Both CT and MRI may be used for intraoperative imaging, although CT is much more commonly accepted.

Cone Beam and Multidetector CT

Cone beam CT (CBCT) imaging has emerged over the last decade as a technology that fulfills the aforementioned criteria. Having gained wide acceptance within the dental and oral surgery fields, CBCT is replacing conventional radiography for in-office diagnosis of periodontal and temporomandibular joint disease.[2] Its applications are expanding into otorhinolaryngology for intraoperative and in-office diagnosis of sino-nasal and otologic disorders. Several commercially available systems are available, including the xCAT ENT (Xoran Technologies, Ann Arbor, Michigan), CereTom (Neurologica, Danvers, Massachusetts), Iluma (Imtec, Ardmore, Oklahoma), and the O-arm (Medtronic, Jacksonville, Florida).

CBCT differs from multidetector CT (MDCT) by its imaging geometry. In conventional MDCT, a narrow fan-shaped beam of radiation is passed through the patient to a detector on a revolving gantry. Data is acquired through slices in the axial plane and an image is created by stacking these images. CBCT, based on volumetric tomography, uses a single diverging cone of radiation that penetrates through the patient and is detected on a 2D area detector. CBCT permits the structure of interest to be imaged within a single rotation. This effectively reduces the time and radiation exposure of image acquisition over MDCT.

CBCT provides better image resolution than MDCT as a function of voxel size and geometry. MDCT relies on rectangular voxels oriented with its longest dimension in the axial plane. Although the surface dimension may approach 0.625 mm, the depth remains in the range of 1 to 2 mm. CBCT resolution is based on isotropic voxels that are equal in all three planes, which permits resolutions as fine as 0.125 mm.[2] Image quality provided by CBCT is quite good. In a study by Hashimoto and colleagues,[3] CBCT was found to produce better image resolution than MDCT for the evaluation of alveolar bone and tooth anatomy when viewed by blinded dental radiologists.

Other benefits of CBCT include easier patient positioning, lower cost, and reduced radiation exposure. MDCT requires the patient to be perpendicular to the x-ray beams within the gantry. Because CBCT creates an image of the entire structural volume, head positioning is not an important factor. The cost of CBCT technology is less than that of MDCT since a motorized mechanism for patient transport through the gantry is not required. The efficiency of the photons with CBCT reduces the heat expenditure within the x-ray tube and reduces the frequency of replacement and maintenance.

CT Devices

Recent advances have reduced the footprint for intraoperative imaging with CT. The intraoperative CT and fluoroscopy units are mobile and can be transported between operating rooms. The xCAT device has dimensions of 32 × 47 × 60 in and weighs approximately 500 lb (**Figs. 1** and **2**). Imaging acquisition occurs at 300 slices in 60 seconds and can obtain a minimum thickness of 0.4 mm. The workstation has the capability of reconstructing triplanar and 3D images.

A similar device is the Iluma scanner, which also acquires images by cone beam tomography and flat panel detection (**Fig. 3**). Ryoo and colleagues[4] demonstrated that the Iluma and miniCAT (in-office version of the xCAT) devices produced images

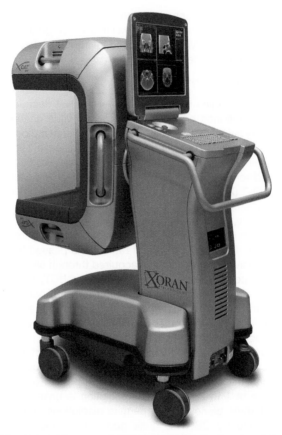

Fig. 1. This portable volume CT scanner (xCAT; Xoran Technologies, Ann Arbor, Michigan) has been optimized for easy use in the operating room. The device has a small footprint for adequate portability and produces images with excellent bony detail. (*Courtesy of* Xoran Technologies, Ann Arbor, MI; with permission.)

of equivalent resolution. The OTOscan device (Neurologica, Danvers, Massachusetts) incorporates multidetector technology, which permits direct coronal imaging and an adjustable scan distance (1–60 cm). The disadvantage is its size, which requires a 9 × 5-ft floor plan. Both the Iluma and OTOscan devices are not configured for use in the operating room. For all CBCT systems, the use of intraoperative CT and fluoroscopy requires that precautions for protecting the patient and operating room staff from ionizing radiation exposure must be in place.

MRI

Intraoperative MRI has been used in the neurosurgery field for over 20 years. Over that time, the technology has evolved to permit the greatest resolution without limiting portability and patient access in the operating room. MRI scanners transmit radiofrequency signals, which are absorbed by protons within the target tissue, and then receives the signals emitted from those protons within the relaxed state. Image quality is proportional to the magnetic field strength. The features of an optimal intraoperative MRI system, including small size to permit portability and open structure to allow access to the patient, conflict with the ability to obtain high-resolution images

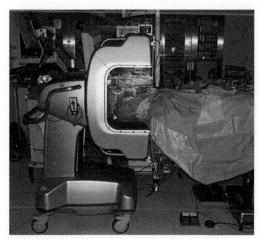

Fig. 2. The xCAT portable volume CT scanner (Xoran Technologies, Ann Arbor, MI) in use during a procedure. The patient's head is positioned within the rotating gantry, which can acquire nearly 300 slices in 60 seconds.

(**Fig. 4**). Intraoperative MRI devices with higher field strengths (1.5 to 3.0 T) permit advanced functionality, including MR angiography, MR venography, diffusion-weighted imaging, and functional MRI. The disadvantage of these systems is that they rule out the use standard surgical instruments near the magnet. This means the patient usually has to be transported into the MRI scanner.

The low field strength (0.15 T) intraoperative MRI systems permit only partial imaging and therefore have limited diagnostic applications.[5] The PoleStar device (Medtronic, Minneapolis, Minnesota) is a low field strength system. Its field of view is approximately 16 × 20 mm.[6] Standard imaging modalities are available with this system including T1, T2, and fluid-attenuated inversion recovery (FLAIR) sequences.

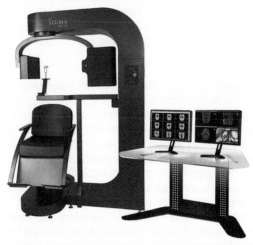

Fig. 3. The Iluma volume CT scanner (Imtec, Ardmore, Oklahoma) occupies about 9 ft by 5 ft of floor space and produces image resolution comparable to that of conventional MDCT. This device is available for use in the office setting as depicted in this image. (*Courtesy of* Imtec, Ardmore, OK; with permission.)

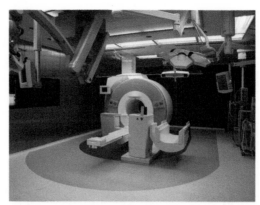

Fig. 4. Intraoperative MRI units require a dedicated operating room, as seen in this example of this intraoperative MRI (BrainLab, Westchester, IL). (*Courtesy of* Jern-Lin Leong, MD, Singapore.)

Scan times range from 8 seconds to 13 minutes with slice thickness between 2 and 8 mm.[6] The PoleStar device offers the benefits of compactness and portability. It weighs approximately 650 kg, making it possible for two people to easily move the device into position.[7] The magnetic gantry consists of two columns spaced approximately 27 cm apart. The gradient coils are mounted on the outside of these columns. The gantry is powered by both electric and hydraulic sources. It can be placed underneath the operating table when not in use during the procedure. The MRI gantry is typically stored within an iron cage when not in use.

The device still requires dedicated operating rooms and instrumentation compatible with the magnetic fields generated by the MRI coils. At this low field strength, however, ferromagnetic instruments can be as close as 25 cm to the coils without attraction.[6] An important safety mechanism is the ability for the closer magnets to attract the instrument and divert it away from the patient's head. Radiofrequency shielding is also required within the operating room to reduce the amount of noise generated by electrical equipment. The entire operating room can be shielded or else a cage can be constructed around the operating room table and device.

Three-dimensional Fluoroscopy

Three-dimensional fluoroscopy is another method of intraoperative imaging that has been implemented in the field of rhinologic surgery. Fluoroscopy has been extensively used in the operating room for orthopedic and vascular procedures. Its portability and maneuverability makes this technology ideal for this application. The patient is placed between the fluoroscope's x-ray source and image intensifier. The x-rays pass through the patient, creating a shadow, which is detected by the image intensifier and video camera. The resulting radiographic image can then be viewed on a portable workstation monitor. New fluoroscopic technology and software have permitted conventional 2D data to be reconstructed into 3D CT-like images. Commercially available products include the OEC 9800 C-arm and FluoroCAT software (GE Healthcare, Lawrence, Massachusetts). The data can then be uploaded onto the InstaTrak workstation (GE Healthcare, Lawrence, Massachusetts) and used as a near real-time update for surgical navigation. A reference array or transmitter is firmly affixed to the patient's head for registration of the device.[8] The C-arm rotates 190° around the patient and captures approximately 200 images, which are reconstructed into triplanar CT images on the image-guided surgery workstation.[9] Similar to CBCT, this imaging modality provides adequate depiction of bony detail with less radiation exposure than that of conventional MDCT. Manarey and Anand[10] showed that the maximal surface radiation dose using the FluoroCAT device was one eighth that of a MDCT scanner.

RATIONALE FOR INTRAOPERATIVE IMAGING

The rationale for intraoperative imaging is based on the rationale for image-guided surgery in endoscopic sinus surgery. Although the nasal telescopes provide brilliant illumination, the endoscopic images are only 2D representations of a complex 3D space. Because the optics of all surgical endoscopes provide a wide-angle view, the images also have spherical distortion around a central point; that is, the images intrinsically have a "fish-eye view." Furthermore the anatomy of interest is surrounded by critical structures. As such, a small amount of perceptual distortion may lead to misperceptions that may direct even a skilled surgeon to a catastrophic complication. Thus, rhinologic surgeons have embraced image-guided surgery as a technological solution for these problems.

Endoscopic techniques are now commonly used for the treatment of complex sino-nasal pathology, including cerebrospinal fluid leak repair, orbital decompression, and pituitary surgery. Recent advances in image-guided surgery and surgical instrumentation are allowing benign and malignant neoplasms of the skull base to be endoscopically managed. Historically, the gold standard for extirpation of skull base neoplasms has been craniofacial resection with a neurosurgical approach. However the morbidity and complications associated with these procedures were quite high, including external facial scars, orbital injury, and alteration of physiologic sinonasal function. Proponents of the open skull base approaches cite an inability to obtain an en bloc resection with endoscopic techniques. Several recent studies have refuted this claim by demonstrating equivalent or lower recurrence rates for those neoplasms resected endoscopically rather than through an open approach. Busquets and Hwang[11] performed a meta-analysis of 700 patients with inverted papilloma treated either endoscopically or nonendoscopically. The recurrence rate in the endoscopic group was 15% compared to 20% in the nonendoscopic control. Sautter and colleagues[12] found a recurrence rate of 22% in those patients with inverted papilloma treated with an endoscopic resection compared to 39% in patients managed with an open approach. Similar results have been obtained with the endoscopic resection of malignant skull base neoplasms. Batra and colleagues[13] observed a recurrence rate of 33% and 36% in patients with anterior skull base tumors treated with a minimally invasive endoscopic resection and craniofacial resection, respectively. Image-guided surgery technology is an important tool for properly identifying the attachment site so that adequate surgery can be performed despite distortions of anatomic landmarks from tumor growth. As intraoperative imaging technology continues to improve, it will have a role in endoscopic skull base surgery to identify residual tumor and ensure a more complete resection.

Image-guided Surgery Developments

Over the last decade, the use of image-guided surgery has significantly increased. Metson[14] looked at the first 1000 procedures incorporating image-guided surgery at his institution and discovered a nearly 74% increase in its usage over the first 2 years. More recently, a survey of 1050 American Rhinologic Society members showed that more than 90% of the participants had routine access to an image-guided surgery system.[15] The goals of image-guided surgery are to reduce the limitations of endoscopic sinus surgery, assist with minimally invasive skull base surgery, and improve patient outcomes. The literature supports the use of image-guided surgery for revision sinus surgery, transsphenoidal hypophysectomies, and even osteoplastic frontal sinus obliteration.[16–19] Fried and colleagues[20] reported a statistically significant reduction in the number of major complications associated with endoscopic sinus surgery when performed with image-guided surgery. These complications included major blood loss, return to the operating room, and abortion of procedure. The patient population in this study was small and other factors that might have contributed to the complications were not discussed. Smith and colleagues[21] performed a systematic review of the literature to determine if image-guided surgery reduced complication rates and improved patient outcomes. The five articles that met the criteria were level 4 (case series) or level 5 (expert opinion) evidence. The conclusion was that sample size and study design preclude randomized trials for the application of this technology. Strauss and colleagues[22] evaluated the practicability of the image-guided surgery technology. The information provided by the image-guided surgery system was felt to be beneficial by 65% of the participating surgeons. In nearly 50% of the uses, the surgical strategy was altered. This was encountered more frequently in less experienced surgeons.

Despite its beneficial role in advanced rhinologic procedure, image-guided surgery does have several limitations. Although the anecdotal reports suggest "submillimetric" accuracy for surgical navigation, in practice the best achievable surgical navigation accuracy (also known as target registration error [TRE]) is probably is 1.5 to 2.0 mm. In select cases, it may be even higher.[23] As a result, image-guided surgery alone may be insufficient for more complex surgical cases. An important limitation is that image-guided surgery is based upon preoperative images and does not reflect anatomic changes from surgical manipulation. Furthermore, surgical navigation accuracy may be compromised by suboptimal registration and, in theory, intraoperative imaging may provide a means for improved registration by enabling the intraoperative placement of fiducial markers.

Intraoperative Imaging for Trauma

An early application of intraoperative imaging was for maxillofacial trauma, specifically the operative repair of orbitozygomatic fractures. Optimal reconstruction involves wide exposure of the fracture segments, reduction with visualization of all fracture sites, and rigid miniplate fixation. Despite meticulous reduction and fixation, ocular symptoms may persist in 30% of the patients and require revision surgery.[24] The benefit of intraoperative imaging would be to eliminate the need for wide exposure and permit manipulation of the fractured segments through less-invasive approaches without an increased requirement for revision surgery. In practice, optimal reduction and fixation of complex fractures often cannot be achieved because, even with exposure provided by today's sophisticated approaches to the craniomaxillofacial skeleton, it remains difficult to reproducibly reduce and fixate fractures in a way that reestablishes preinjury contours, projection, and symmetry (**Fig. 5**). In concept, intraoperative imaging would provide an intraoperative means for assessing the adequacy of fracture reduction. Several studies evaluated the use of intraoperative CT to determine the need for a further reduction of fracture segments and found the rate to be approximately 20%.[25,26]

CLINICAL REPORTS OF INTRAOPERATIVE IMAGING

Applications of intraoperative imaging in rhinology are gaining interest as a means for compensating for the well-recognized limitations of image-guided surgery. The aim of

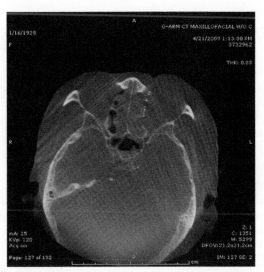

Fig. 5. This intraoperative axial CT, obtained with the O-arm (Medtronic, Jacksonville, FL), shows an implant along the left medial orbital wall. The implant is adequately placed to prevent the herniation of orbital contents into the ethmoid region. (*Courtesy of* Parul Goyal, MD, Syracuse, NY.)

intraoperative imaging is to provide near real-time imaging during advanced rhinologic procedures. Cone beam technology has permitted CT scanners to become the intraoperative imaging modality of choice. Several early studies looked at the technical feasibility of using intraoperative CT scanners. Das and colleagues[27] evaluated several parameters involved in the setup of the xCAT device. They found improved accuracy of the image-guided surgery system after updating it with intraoperative images. The mean amount of time involved with image acquisition and uploading into the image-guided surgery hardware was 13 minutes. The Xoran scanner was compatible with all commercially available image-guided surgery systems. Wise and colleagues[28] found that physicians in training more accurately identified sinonasal anatomy when performing endoscopic sinus dissections with both image-guided surgery and intraoperative imaging than with image-guided surgery alone.

More recently, the clinical utility of intraoperative imaging and its impact on surgical decision-making has been studied. Jackman and colleagues[29] performed intraoperative volume CT scans on 20 patients undergoing functional endoscopic sinus surgery. In this report, 30% of these patients required further surgical manipulation—a surgical decision based purely on the images provided by intraoperative imaging. Reasons for the altered surgical plan included residual uncinate process, incomplete removal of type III frontoethmoid cells, and retained ethmoid partitions. In a similar study, Batra and colleagues[30] found that intraoperative CT resulted in 24% of the patients requiring refinement in their sinus procedures. The information obtained from the intraoperative image led to a more extensive ethmoid dissection, frontal stent repositioning (**Fig. 6**), further tumor resection (**Figs. 7** and **8**), and alteration of a Draf IIb.

As an extension of neurosurgical applications, intraoperative MRI has been used during the endoscopic resection of sellar lesions. Anand and colleagues[31] reported their experience with this intraoperative technology and concluded that endoscopy and intraoperative MRI provided complementary information. In this report, 2 of 10 patients required re-resection of their pituitary adenoma based on intraoperative

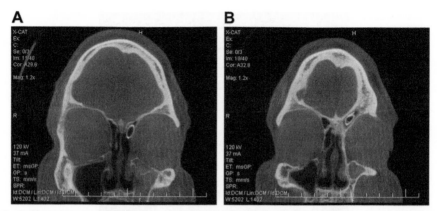

Fig. 6. These intraoperative coronal CT images, obtained with the xCAT (Xoran Technologies, Ann Arbor, MI) show a frontal sinus stent placed during revision endoscopic frontal sinusotomy. The intraoperative CT was used to confirm proper placement of the stent in the left frontal recess (A) and sinus (B).

imaging. However, 2 of 10 patients had evidence of residual tumor on MRI, but normal repeat endoscopy indicating no further surgical intervention. A significant disadvantage was the interference between the MRI magnet and the video monitor. The monitor had to be placed at least 4 ft away from the MRI gantry.

Fluoroscopy has been extensively used as an intraoperative imaging modality in orthopedic and vascular surgery. Three-dimensional reconstructions created from the data acquired by the fluoroscope have been used to provide near real-time updates of image-guided surgery platforms during endoscopic sinus surgery. Brown and colleagues[9] evaluated the use of the FluoroCAT device on 14 consecutive patients undergoing image-guided endoscopic sinus surgery. With experience, the FluoroCAT provided adequate resolution of bony anatomy. The image quality was adversely affected by nasal packing, blood within the paranasal sinuses, and

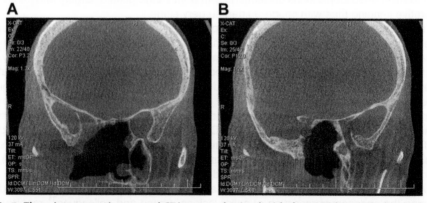

Fig. 7. These intraoperative coronal CT images, obtained with the xCAT (Xoran Technologies, Ann Arbor, MI) show the maxillary, ethmoid (A) and sphenoid (B) cavities after the endoscopic resection of a recurrent squamous cell carcinoma. The intraoperative CT was used to assess the adequacy of the resection as well as the extent of bony dissection.

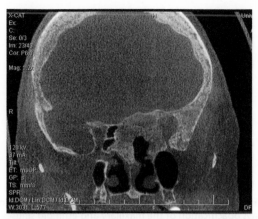

Fig. 8. This intraoperative coronal CT image, obtained with the xCAT (Xoran Technologies, Ann Arbor, MI), demonstrates a partial resection of a fibro-osseous tumor of the sphenoeth-moid region. At this stage of the procedure, a large of amount bony tissue had been removed from the ethmoid with the drill. After review of this image, additional work was performed to drill additional bone from sphenoid bone itself.

polyposis. They concluded that further evidence is required to define indications for this intraoperative technology.

DISADVANTAGES OF INTRAOPERATIVE IMAGING

As CT imaging modalities become more accessible, more thought must be given toward issues of radiation exposure and patient safety. Medical imaging accounts for nearly 11% of a person's lifetime exposure to radiation.[32] Approximately 62 million CT scans are performed each year, up from 3 million in 1980.[32,33] The reasons for this substantial increase include the shorter scan time, increased usage in the pediatric population, and its expanding role in preventative medicine. A significant amount of information regarding radiation-induced malignancies has been collected by studying atomic bomb survivors. A linear occurrence of solid cancers has been noted with exposures between 100 and 4000 mSv.[32] Before 2001, there were a predicted 700 deaths per year as a result of radiation exposure from CT head examinations. The same study showed nearly 500 deaths attributable to CT imaging in those patients less than 15 years of age.[32] The risk of developing a radiation-induced malignancy over one's lifetime increased exponentially with decreasing age of exposure. This information has forced the medical field to adopt the principle of using the lowest possible radiation dose. Advancing technology and an ability to adjust CT parameters have permitted lower radiation exposure, especially in the pediatric population.[34] Current CBCT scanners are capable of acquiring images with adequate resolution with scan times of 20 seconds and effective radiation doses of approximately 0.08 mSv.[35]

In addition to increasing overall risk of carcinogenesis, sinus CT imaging can lead to injuries of surrounding organs, specifically to the lens of the eye and to the parotid gland. Historically, radiation doses of 500 to 2000 mGy were shown to induce the onset of cataracts and parotitis. Bassim and colleagues[36] measured the radiation exposure of a MDCT at the lens and parotid gland to be 29.5 mGy and 30 mGy respectively. Research has shown that radiation exposure from CBCT is one ninth that from

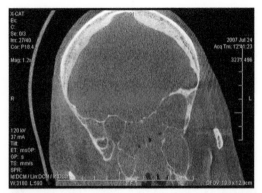

Fig. 9. This intraoperative coronal CT image, obtained with the xCAT (Xoran Technologies, Ann Arbor, MI), shows opacification of the maxillary and ethmoid sinuses with blood. There is some heterogeneity within the maxillary sinus, suggesting the presence of blood. The completeness of the ethmoid dissection is marked by the lack of bony partitions. However, the blood within the sinuses creates the illusion of residual disease.

conventional MDCT.[2] Das and colleagues[27] measured the radiation exposure of the xCAT at the lens and orbital apex as compared to that for MDCT controls. The exposure was two to four times less with the xCAT.

The image resolution of volume-rendering CT scanners is equivalent to that of the MDCT devices for bony anatomy. However, a limitation of the CBCT technology is some loss in the quality of soft tissue imaging. Fluid within the dissected sinus cavity may be confused for edematous mucosa, polyps, and retained secretions and blood (**Fig. 9**) or even residual tumor (**Fig. 10**). It is important in these situations to remember that intraoperative imaging is a tool that provides complementary information to the endoscopic portion of the procedure. Any suspicious findings on the intraoperative CT must be evaluated endoscopically.

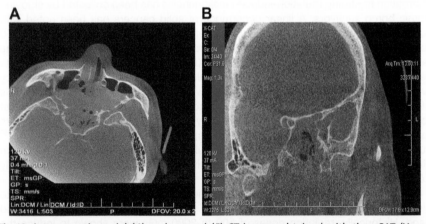

Fig. 10. Intraoperative axial (*A*) and coronal (*B*) CT images obtained with the xCAT (Xoran Technologies, Ann Arbor, MI) after resection of a large clival chordoma. The blood within the sphenoid sinus prevents optimal assessment of tumor resection, but the bony detail on the imaging confirms the extent of the bony dissection.

Because intraoperative imaging is new technology, many costs are associated with its use. Prices for an intraoperative volume CT scanner are approximately $300,000 (or more) and an intraoperative MRI ranges from $1 million to $7 million, depending on the field strength. Other costs include training the operating room staff and the extra operative time to manipulate the system. The setup time required to rescan the patient, process the images, and often reregister the image-guided surgery system averages between 13 and 45 minutes.[25,27] The goal of intraoperative imaging, however, is to permit more successful minimally invasive surgeries, which should effectively reduce the patient's length of hospital stay and need for revision surgery. Hall and Truwit[5] found that the length of stay was 55% shorter in those resections performed with intraoperative MRI guidance. Total hospital costs were subsequently 14% lower. Further studies are required to fully define the overall cost of this technology.

SUMMARY

The application of endoscopic techniques has expanded beyond the treatment of inflammatory sinus disease toward the resection of anterior and middle skull base lesions. Image-guided surgery has emerged as an important tool that compensates for the limitations of surgical endoscopy. The disadvantage of image-guided surgery, however, is its dependence on preoperative imaging data. Intraoperative imaging provides near real-time imaging that has the potential to improve surgical outcomes and reduce operative morbidity. Its application in the fields of neurosurgery and maxillofacial trauma has shown a distinct benefit with a lower incidence of revision surgery. The role of intraoperative imaging in endoscopic sinus and skull base surgery has demonstrated great promise in recent literature. It has had an impact on surgical decision-making during functional endoscopic sinus surgery and the resection of anterior skull base neoplasia. Advances in portable MRI and volumetric CT technology have enhanced the efficiency and safety of intraoperative imaging. Although further studies are required to quantify the precise utility of this new technology, it appears that intraoperative imaging will be an important tool for rhinologic surgery.

REFERENCES

1. International Society for Computer-Aided Surgery. Goals and missions of ISCAS. Available at: http://www.iscas.net. Accessed July 15, 2009.
2. White SC. Cone-beam imaging in dentistry. Health Phys 2008;95(5):628–37.
3. Hashimoto K, Arai Y, Iwai K, et al. A comparison of a new limited cone beam computed tomography machine for dental use with a multidetector row helical CT machine. Oral Surg Oral Med Oral Pathol Oral Radiol Endod 2003;95(3): 371–7.
4. Ryoo C, Barin K, Karanfilov B. Comparison of cone beam computed tomography versus helical high resolution computed tomography. Columbus (OH): The Ohio State University Medical Center; 2008.
5. Hall WA, Truwit CL. Intraoperative MR-guided neurosurgery. J Magn Reson Imaging 2008;27(2):368–75.
6. Ntoukas V, Krishnan R, Seifert V. The new generation PoleStar n20 for conventional neurosurgical operating rooms: a preliminary report. Neurosurgery 2008; 62(3 Suppl 1):82–9 [discussion: 89–90].
7. Seifert V. Intraoperative MRI in neurosurgery: technical overkill or the future of brain surgery? Neurol India 2003;51(3):329–32.
8. Kahler DM. Image guidance: fluoroscopic navigation. Clin Orthop Relat Res 2004;421:70–6.

9. Brown SM, Sadoughi B, Cuellar H, et al. Feasibility of near real-time image-guided sinus surgery using intraoperative fluoroscopic computed axial tomography. Otolaryngol Head Neck Surg 2007;136(2):268–73.

10. Manarey CR, Anand VK. Radiation dosimetry of the FluoroCAT scan for real-time endoscopic sinus surgery. Otolaryngol Head Neck Surg 2006;135(3):409–12.

11. Busquets JM, Hwang PH. Endoscopic resection of sinonasal inverted papilloma: a meta-analysis. Otolaryngol Head Neck Surg 2006;134(3):476–82.

12. Sautter NB, Cannady SB, Citardi MJ, et al. Comparison of open versus endoscopic resection of inverted papilloma. Am J Rhinol 2007;21(3):320–3.

13. Batra PS, Citardi MJ, Worley S, et al. Resection of anterior skull base tumors: comparison of combined traditional and endoscopic techniques. Am J Rhinol 2005;19(5):521–8.

14. Metson R. Image-guided sinus surgery: lessons learned from the first 1000 cases. Otolaryngol Head Neck Surg 2003;128(1):8–13.

15. Orlandi RR, Petersen E. Image guidance: a survey of attitudes and use. Am J Rhinol 2006;20(4):406–11.

16. Chiu AG, Vaughan WC. Revision endoscopic frontal sinus surgery with surgical navigation. Otolaryngol Head Neck Surg 2004;130(3):312–8.

17. Jagannathan J, Prevedello DM, Ayer VS, et al. Computer-assisted frameless stereotaxy in transsphenoidal surgery at a single institution: review of 176 cases. Neurosurg Focus 2006;20(2):E9.

18. Sindwani R, Metson R. Impact of image guidance on complications during osteoplastic frontal sinus surgery. Otolaryngol Head Neck Surg 2004;131(3):150–5.

19. Innis W, Byrne P, Tufano RP. Image-guided osteoplastic frontal sinusotomy. Am J Rhinol 2005;19(5):430–4.

20. Fried MP, Moharir VM, Shin J, et al. Comparison of endoscopic sinus surgery with and without image guidance. Am J Rhinol 2002;16(4):193–7.

21. Smith TL, Stewart MG, Orlandi RR, et al. Indications for image-guided sinus surgery: the current evidence. Am J Rhinol 2007;21(1):80–3.

22. Strau G, Koulechov K, Rottger S, et al. Evaluation of a navigation system for ENT with surgical efficiency criteria. Laryngoscope 2006;116(4):564–72.

23. Citardi MJ, Batra PS. Intraoperative surgical navigation for endoscopic sinus surgery: rationale and indications. Curr Opin Otolaryngol Head Neck Surg 2007;15(1):23–7.

24. Kwon JH, Kim JG, Moon JH, et al. Clinical analysis of surgical approaches for orbital floor fractures. Arch Facial Plast Surg 2008;10(1):21–4.

25. Stanley RB Jr. Use of intraoperative computed tomography during repair of orbitozygomatic fractures. Arch Facial Plast Surg 1999;1(1):19–24.

26. Hoelzle F, Klein M, Schwerdtner O, et al. Intraoperative computed tomography with the mobile CT Tomoscan M during surgical treatment of orbital fractures. Int J Oral Maxillofac Surg 2001;30(1):26–31.

27. Das S, Maeso PA, Figueroa RE, et al. The use of portable intraoperative computed tomography scanning for real-time image guidance: a pilot cadaver study. Am J Rhinol 2008;22(2):166–9.

28. Wise SK, Harvey RJ, Goddard JC, et al. Combined image guidance and intraoperative computed tomography in facilitating endoscopic orientation within and around the paranasal sinuses. Am J Rhinol 2008;22(6):635–41.

29. Jackman AH, Palmer JN, Chiu AG, et al. Use of intraoperative CT scanning in endoscopic sinus surgery: a preliminary report. Am J Rhinol 2008;22(2):170–4.

30. Batra PS, Kanowitz SJ, Citardi MJ. Clinical utility of intraoperative volume computed tomography scanner for endoscopic sinonasal and skull base procedures. Am J Rhinol 2008;22(5):511–5.

31. Anand VK, Schwartz TH, Hiltzik DH, et al. Endoscopic transphenoidal pituitary surgery with real-time intraoperative magnetic resonance imaging. Am J Rhinol 2006;20(4):401–5.

32. Brenner DJ, Hall EJ. Computed tomography—an increasing source of radiation exposure. N Engl J Med 2007;357(22):2277–84.

33. Amis ES Jr, Butler PF, Applegate KE, et al. American College of Radiology white paper on radiation dose in medicine. J Am Coll Radiol 2007;4(5):272–84.

34. Donnelly LF, Emery KH, Brody AS, et al. Minimizing radiation dose for pediatric body applications of single-detector helical CT: strategies at a large children's hospital. AJR Am J Roentgenol 2001;176(2):303–6.

35. Zoumalan RA, Lebowitz RA, Wang E, et al. Flat panel cone beam computed tomography of the sinuses. Otolaryngol Head Neck Surg 2009;140(6):841–4.

36. Bassim MK, Ebert CS, Sit RC, et al. Radiation dose to the eyes and parotids during CT of the sinuses. Otolaryngol Head Neck Surg 2005;133(4):531–3.

Innovations in Microdebrider Technology and Design

Seth Bruggers, MD, Raj Sindwani, MD, FACS, FRCS(C)*

KEYWORDS

- Microdebrider • Powered instrumentation
- Endoscopic sinus surgery • Inferior turbinate reduction
- Vacuum rotary dissector

Techniques in endoscopic sinus surgery (ESS) have continued to evolve, often propelled forward by technological advances in instrumentation. The microdebrider is one of the premier innovations in instrumentation for ESS. The use of this instrument has continued to grow more popular in recent years and has reduced reliance on traditional nonpowered sinus instruments, such as curettes and forceps. Microdebriders are preferred for ESS by many surgeons because the instruments spare adjacent mucosa during surgery and offer improved precision, more expeditious tissue removal, and better visualization.[1–3]

The original design for what we now know as the microdebrider was patented by Urban in 1969 as a "vacuum rotary dissector." It was initially used by the House group in the 1970s for morselizing acoustic neuromas, but later became more widely used in orthopedic surgery for arthroscopy. These devices were introduced for nasal surgery in 1994 by Setliff[4] and Parsons,[5] and successive models have appeared with improved design and versatility.[6] The microdebrider is a cylindrical, electrically powered shaver supplied with continuous suction.[7] The basic design consists of a hollow shaft with a rotating or oscillating inner cannula. Applied suction draws soft tissue into a port on the side of the tip when it is open and, as the blade rotates or oscillates back, the trapped tissue is sheared off between the inner and outer cannulas. The slower the speed of the inner blade, the larger the tissue bites are, as more tissue is able to be suctioned into the port before being cut off. Thus the faster the blade speed, the less aggressive the instrument.

The morselized pieces are small enough to be sucked down the instrument, aided by self-irrigating hand pieces, which provide a steady stream of saline through a separate set of tubing. Although individual pieces are small, the histology of the tissue is well preserved and tissue removal by microdebrider has been shown to be no different

Department of Otolaryngology—Head & Neck Surgery, St Louis University School of Medicine, 6th Floor FDT, 3635 Vista Avenue at Grand Boulevard, St Louis, MO 63110, USA
* Corresponding author.
E-mail address: sindwani@slu.edu (R. Sindwani).

Otolaryngol Clin N Am 42 (2009) 781–787
doi:10.1016/j.otc.2009.07.003
0030-6665/09/$ – see front matter © 2009 Elsevier Inc. All rights reserved.

than piecemeal resection using conventional instrumentation with regards to pathologic examination.[8]

Most microdebrider hand pieces have maintained the basic cylindrical design. These hand pieces are usually held as one would hold a scalpel, although some, such as the Diego microdebrider (Gyrus ACMI-ENT Division, Bartlett, Tennessee) have a pistol-grip design, which some consider more ergonomic. Ultimately, the choice of hand piece becomes a matter of surgeon comfort and preference, as the various microdebriders available are materially similar with respect to function.

With the proliferation of image-guidance systems for ESS, there was growing interest in being able to also track the end of a microdebrider during complex cases to minimize the number of movements required to establish and maintain surgical orientation. Optical-based navigation systems responded with "universal calibration" paradigms, which permit the navigation of virtually any rigid instrument by affixing an array of reflective spheres to the desired instrument. Some microdebrider manufacturers have also recently modified hand-piece designs to include a post that quickly couples with the hardware necessary for image-guided surgery calibration (**Fig. 1**).

MICRODEBRIDER BLADES

Various blade configurations have been developed for the microdebrider. The edges on both the inner and outer cannulas can be either straight-edged or serrated. The serrated edges allow for better gripping of soft tissue, while straight edges are less traumatic and more sparing of adjacent tissue (**Fig. 2**).

Depending on the relative angles of the openings to the inner and outer cannulas, the cutting action can either be a guillotine or scissors action. Most microdebrider blades have a scissors-type action, with an angle between the openings of the inner and outer cannulas allowing for a traveling plane of resection, so that the shearing force is only applied to a small area of tissue at a time, maximizing efficiency. With a guillotine mechanism, the apertures of the two cannulas run parallel to one another and the entire bite of tissue is sheared off at once.

Blades can be set to rotate or oscillate. Oscillation typically runs at a slower speed (up to 5000 rpm) and is beneficial in soft tissue resection. At slower speeds, the port

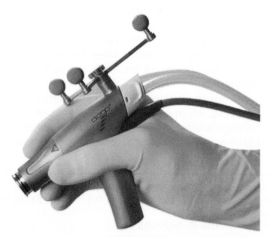

Fig.1. Diego microdebrider (*From* Gyrus ACMI-ENT Division, Bartlett, Tennessee; with permission.) equipped with built-in post for fixation of reflective spheres array from an optical-based image-guidance system. (*From* BrainLab AG, Munich, Germany; with permission.)

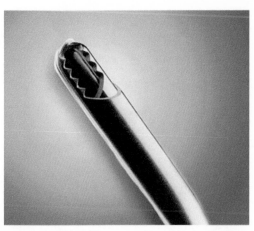

Fig. 2. A microdebrider tip with serrated outer and inner cannulas. (*From* Medtronic-Xomed, Jacksonville, Florida; with permission.)

remains open longer, allowing more soft tissue to be drawn into the aperture before the cut is made. Forward and reverse settings are faster (up to 15,000 rpm) and allow a drill-like action more suitable for takedown of thicker bone, such as during takedown of the maxillary crest during septoplasty or septal spur resection, or during dacryocystorhinostomy. However, due to their relatively low revolution speed, these instruments are less efficient at removing thick bone compared with high-speed drills.

Newer microdebrider designs permit the shaver blade to be rotated on their primary axis to orient the aperture toward the tissue to be removed. Microdebrider blades are also available with a variety of prebent angles, with either a concave or convex bend (**Fig. 3**). This allows improved access to some hard-to-reach areas, such as the paranasal sinuses, though these bent cannulas do tend to be more prone to clogging than straight cannulas. Some, such as the Straightshot M4 (Medtronic-Xomed, Jacksonville, Florida) (**Fig. 4**), are prebent but also allow 360° tip rotation, accomplished by a wheel on the handpiece.[9] Products of other manufacturers offer similar capabilities.

Specialty microdebrider blades are made for specific tasks. The inferior turbinate blade is a small-diameter blade (available in 2.0- and 2.9-mm sizes) and has a beveled guard on the back of the blade to dissect and then protect the turbinate mucosa while performing submucous resection of the vascular erectile tissue (**Fig. 5**). Studies have

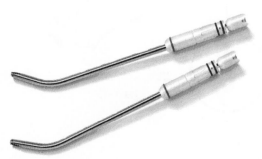

Fig. 3. Prebent blades are available in a variety of angles, with different port orientations allowing access to different parts of the nasal cavity and paranasal sinuses.

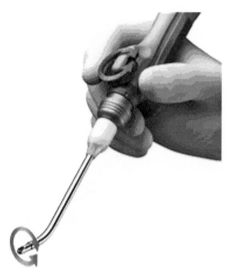

Fig. 4. The Straightshot M4 (Medtronic-Xomed, Jacksonville, Florida), an example of a microdebrider tip with independent blade and tip rotation.

demonstrated that, by sparing the surface respiratory epithelium, less crusting and synechiae formation occur postoperation than when cautery is used. Also, incidence of osteitis of the concha is lower.[10,11] The edged tip available in some microdebriders is also sharp enough to make the initial stab incision through which a plane of dissection may be created along the length of the turbinate. Another example of a specialized blade is the Radenoid blade (Medtronic-Xomed, Jacksonville, Florida), which is tailored for removal of adenoid tissue, although suction electrocautery is typically needed afterwards for control of bleeding in the adenoid bed.

THE MICRODEBRIDER AND BLEEDING

The real advantage of the microdebrider comes from its ability to continuously suction away blood and fragments of tissue and bone. Given the small operative field in ESS,

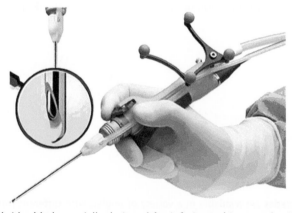

Fig. 5. Microdebrider blade specially designed for inferior turbinate reduction.

even a small amount of bleeding can significantly impair visibility during surgery. Using conventional instrumentation, the surgeon is constantly alternating between instruments for taking down tissue and a suction cannula for clearing the field before the next tissue manipulation. The ability to simultaneously suction blood away from the surgical field is especially advantageous during ESS for nasal polyps, given the propensity of polypoid tissue to bleed during removal. The microdebrider allows the surgeon to continue to work much longer with no sacrifice of visibility and without the time lost by repeatedly switching instruments.

Significant bleeding intraoperatively can increase the risk of complications and may even force premature termination of the procedure. Despite the robust proliferation of microdebriders and their effectiveness at continuously clearing blood from the field, current models have a major shortcoming: They do nothing to actually reduce bleeding.

Recent advances in microdebrider technology now permit the added ability to control bleeding while retaining the shaving and suctioning capabilities of conventional microdebriders. The PK Diego (Gyrus ACMI-ENT Division, Bartlett, Tennessee) **(Fig. 6)** has the ability to also provide hemostasis by delivering bipolar energy to the end of its blade. The blade is surrounded by layers of insulation sandwiching inner and outer electrodes. The instrument can be set to low (10 W), medium (20 W), or high (40 W) power. A drawback to the current model is that it has a fairly small zone of bipolar cautery, which is located at the distal aspect of the blade, perpendicular to the suction aperture. Ideally the two poles would be on opposite sides of the aperture, allowing for more effective hemostasis at the site of (and perhaps even during) actual tissue removal. A recent prospective, controlled study of 80 patients undergoing surgery for chronic rhinosinusitis with polyps found that the use of the bipolar-equipped PK Diego was associated with significantly less blood loss and shorter operative times compared with surgery performed using a conventional microdebrider.[12] The fact that the PK Diego functions using bipolar energy as opposed to monopolar is significant, as this limits the transmission of heat to adjacent intraorbital and intracranial structures. The application of this instrument is also well suited for submucosal inferior turbinate reduction where bleeding from the turbinate interior as well as the entry site can be controlled, and for endonasal removal of vascularized tissues (adenoids or tumors). The PK Diego is the only microdebrider currently available that offers a means of hemostasis in addition to the shaving and suctioning features common to this class of instrument.

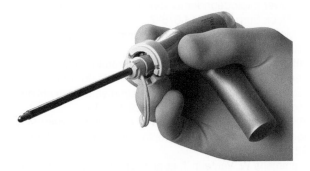

Fig. 6. The PK Diego (Gyrus ACMI-ENT Division, Bartlett, Tennessee) which uses bipolar energy to achieve hemostasis. (*From* Gyrus ACMI-ENT Division, Bartlett, Tennessee; with permission.)

LIMITATIONS OF MICRODEBRIDERS

Like any other instrument, microdebriders have certain limitations that must be recognized if these tools are to be used effectively and safely. Microdebriders operate at the relatively slow speed of 15,000 rpm, as opposed to high-speed drills, which operate at around 80,000 rpm, making them far less efficient at removing significant amounts of thick bone. Microdebriders are also heavier than conventional instruments and are electrically powered. This means that the tactile feedback component of surgery is markedly diminished with microdebriders. The lack of tactile feedback is most pronounced during soft tissue removal, and less so with bony applications.

The powered nature of these instruments and their use in a confined space in close proximity to the skull base and orbit have raised concerns about the safety of these tools in ESS. Bhatti and colleagues[13] described two cases of ocular injury, one resulting in restrictive ophthalmoplegia and another in transection of the medial rectus. In both cases, it was argued that the strong suction of the microdebrider allowed orbital fat or even extraocular muscles to be pulled through a relatively small defect in the lamina paprycea, leading to subsequent injury by the rapidly moving blade. Berenholz and colleagues[14] described a case of subarachnoid hemorrhage after functional ESS using the microdebrider, also thought to be caused by the strength of suction. It behooves the surgeon using the microdebrider to bear in mind that, although major complications from ESS are fortunately rare,[15] complications that do occur when a microdebrider is employed tend to progress more quickly because of the powered nature and suction of this device. Finally, the use of microdebrider incurs expense. The costs associated with the use of a microdebrider include the capital expense of the system and ongoing costs of the disposable blades. The various blades available range in price.

SUMMARY

Microdebriders represent an important advance in surgical rhinology. The use of microdebriders for ESS offers marked advantages, including mucosal preservation, improved precision, expeditious tissue removal, and better visualization. Microdebrider design and technology have continued to improve. These powered instruments have limitations that must be understood to avoid complications related to their use.

REFERENCES

1. Christmas DA, Krouse JH. Powered instrumentation in functional endoscopic sinus surgery I: surgical technique. Ear Nose Throat J 1996;75:33–40.
2. Goode RL. Power microdebrider for functional endoscopic sinus surgery. Otolaryngol Head Neck Surg 1996;114:676–7.
3. Hamels K, Morre TD, Clement PA. The hummer, shaver or microdebrider. Acta Otorhinolaryngol Belg 1997;51:89–91.
4. Setliff RC III. The hummer: a remedy for apprehension in functional endoscopic sinus surgery. Otolaryngol Clin North Am 1996;29:95–104.
5. Parsons DS. Rhinologic uses of powered instrumentation in children beyond sinus surgery. Otolaryngol Clin North Am 1996;29:105–14.
6. Chandra RK, Schlosser R, Kennedy DW. Use of the 70 degree diamond burr in the management of complicated frontal sinus disease. Laryngoscope 2004; 114:188–92.
7. Sauer M, Lemmens W, Vauterin T, et al. Comparing the microdebrider and standard instruments in endoscopic sinus surgery: a double-blind randomized study. B-ENT 2007;3:1–7.

8. Zweig JL, Schaitkin BM, Fan CY. Histopathology of tissue samples removed using microdebrider technique: implications for endoscopic sinus surgery. Am J Rhinol 2000;14:27–32.
9. Bumm K, Wurm J, Bohr C, et al. New endoscopic instruments for paranasal sinus surgery. Otolaryngol Head Neck Surg 2005;133(3):444–9.
10. Joniau S, Wong I, Rajapaksa S, et al. Long term comparison between submucosal cauterization and powered reduction of inferior turbinates. Laryngoscope 2006;116(9):1612–6.
11. Friedman M, Tanyeri H, Lim J, et al. A safe, alternative technique for inferior turbinate reduction. Laryngoscope 1999;109:1834–7.
12. Kumar N, Sindwani R. Bipolar microdebrider reduces operative time and blood loss during nasal polyp surgery. Laryngoscope 2009;119–43.
13. Bhatti MT, Giannoni CM, Raynor E, et al. Ocular motility complications after endoscopic sinus surgery with powered cutting instruments. Otolaryngol Head Neck Surg 2001;125:501–9.
14. Berenholz L, Kessler A, Sarfaty S, et al. Subarachnoid hemorrhage: a complication of endoscopic sinus surgery using powered instrumentation. Otolaryngol Head Neck Surg 1999;121:665–7.
15. Dalziel K, Stein K, Ali Rould, et al. Endoscopic sinus surgery for the excision of nasal polyposis: a systematic review of safety and effectiveness. Am J Rhinol 2006;20:506–19.

Evolving Trends in Powered Endoscopic Sinus Surgery

Seth Bruggers, MD, Raj Sindwani, MD, FACS, FRCS(C)*

KEYWORDS

- Powered sinus surgery • Suction-irrigation drill • Coblation
- Ultrasonic aspirator • Sonopet Omni • CUSA NXT
- Endoscopic sinus instruments

The introduction of the rigid nasal endoscope for the diagnosis and surgical management of sinonasal disorders is the single greatest advance in rhinology to date. Endoscopy provided improved visualization of sinonasal anatomy and pioneered the way for sinus surgery to safely extend beyond the nasal cavity and paranasal sinuses.[1] However, with one hand occupied holding the endoscope, the surgeon is left with only one free hand with which to operate. A logical development from this reality is a need for surgical instruments that could perform a variety of tasks at once. In addition, the desire of endoscopic surgeons to access different regions of the adjacent intracranial cavity and orbit necessitated the development of tools that permitted the safe removal of significant amounts of bone in a controlled and expeditious manner.

Powered sinus instruments entered the landscape several decades ago, with the introduction of the microdebrider. Since then, several other powered tools, such as the endoscopic drill (equipped with suction-irrigation), coblator, and the ultrasonic aspirator have been used during endoscopic sinus and skull base surgery. As with the microdebrider, these innovations may also one day become a mainstay of the rhinologist's arsenal. The primary drawback of powered instruments over conventional tools continues to be the higher costs associated with their use, which include the initial capital expenditure for the system and ongoing costs of disposable blades, bits, tips, and tubing. It should be noted that the effective use of powered instrumentation requires an intimate understanding of the capabilities and limitations of these instruments. In contradistinction to conventional instrumentation, powered tools, by definition, have an electrical supply enabling them to move very rapidly and are often equipped with continuous suction. This has raised concerns over the potential for the

Disclosures and conflicts of interest: none.
Department of Otolaryngology–Head and Neck Surgery, St Louis University, 6th Floor FDT, 3635 Vista Avenue at Grand Boulevard, St Louis, MO 63110, USA
* Corresponding author.
E-mail address: sindwani@slu.edu (R. Sindwani).

Otolaryngol Clin N Am 42 (2009) 789–798
doi:10.1016/j.otc.2009.08.016
0030-6665/09/$ – see front matter © 2009 Elsevier Inc. All rights reserved.

oto.theclinics.com

rapid escalation of complications, if and when they occur. It should be underscored, however, that these are still tools nonetheless, and they are not in and of themselves more or less dangerous, provided the operator possesses the requisite surgical experience and understanding of both the disease process and the tools selected to modify it.

ENDOSCOPIC DRILLS

Endoscopic drills are far less commonly used than the microdebrider, given that the microdebrider is able to effectively handle the thin bony partitions of the ethmoid that are addressed with most endoscopic sinus procedures. Where the bone is thicker than microdebrider blades can handle, a variety of drills and drill bits have been developed for endoscopic use. Conventional instruments can sometimes be used in cases requiring significant bony removal, but the greater force needed to take down thick bone can result in poorly controlled movements that risk injury. The advantage of drills in this setting is that they permit expeditious and more controlled bony removal.

Technology

Unlike the more familiar otologic drills, drills intended for endoscopic use ideally have a slimmer profile permitting them to be passed readily into and out of the nostrils. They also often have a protective sheath that protects tissues from the posterior aspect of the drill burr and are equipped with continuous suction and irrigation functions (**Fig. 1**). A significant drawback to the sheaths, however, is that they do increase the diameter of the drill and thus contribute to decreased visualization of the already narrow surgical field. The advantages and disadvantages of the guarded drills must be reconciled depending on the details of the case and the anatomic configuration encountered.

With all drills, the number of flutes on the burr determines how aggressively the drill will function. Fewer flutes will result in faster and more aggressive takedown of bone, but often at the expense of control. Increasing the speed of rotation also provides more rapid removal of bone, although in this case there is actually improved control with a faster spinning burr. Diamond burrs are much less aggressive than cutting burrs in general and are available for smoothing bone edges, although these tend to be much slower at takedown of bone than cutting burrs. This makes them the better

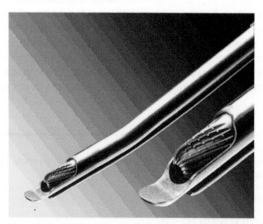

Fig. 1. Suction-irrigation endoscopic drill displaying a cutting burr with protective back sheath. (*Courtesy of* Medtronic Xomed, Jacksonville, FL; with permission.)

choice where a longer operative time is a worthwhile price to pay to minimize risks of damage to delicate surrounding structures. Endoscopic drills also have built-in suction to constantly remove blood and debris and thus allow for improved visibility. This is a very valuable feature.

Clinical Applications

Drills are not needed for routine endoscopic sinus surgery. However, they can be very beneficial for more advanced techniques that require the removal of thicker bone. A variety of clinical scenarios and procedures may be augmented with the use of high-speed drills. Perhaps the most common application of drills is in surgery of the frontal sinus. After conservative measures aimed at widening the frontal recess fail, more aggressive techniques targeting the frontal sinus ostium and the floor of the sinus are pursued.[2] The frontal ostium is located in the posteromedial aspect of the thick floor and can be enlarged unilaterally or bilaterally using a drill. The high-speed drill is effective at resecting the floor and nasofrontal beak region and maybe used to create a large common aperture that drains both frontal sinuses via the endoscopic modified Lothrop procedure (EMLP; also known as the Draf III or bilateral frontal drill-out procedure) (**Fig. 2**). This technique was described by Draf[3] and others[4,5] and involves resection of both frontal sinus floors and interfrontal septum through a superior septectomy. A meta-analysis of the EMLP demonstrated that in experienced hands, this technique is very effective in the management of refractory frontal sinus disease and is associated with a low rate of complications (<1% major and 4% minor complication rates).[6] During this procedure, drilling proceeds from the frontal ostium anteriorly through the frontal floor and nasofrontal beak area, and great care must be taken to avoid trauma to the skull base and anterior ethmoidal artery, which constitute the posterior boundary of the dissection. The burr guard available on some endoscopic drills may be of considerable value when drilling out the frontal sinus, where damage to the posterior aspect of the ostium and recess can lead to unwanted mucosal trauma and resultant stenosis or possibly even intracranial injury.

The proliferation of endoscopic transsphenoidal approaches to the sella and beyond have created novel clinical situations that require the controlled removal of bone from virtually all aspects of the sphenoid sinus, beginning at the face for initial access, through the posterior and superior walls toward the clivus and sellar regions, and laterally for decompression of the optic nerve.[7–9] Suction-irrigation drills are important during these procedures not only to continuously evacuate blood and debris

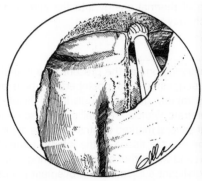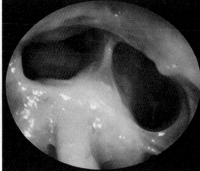

Fig. 2. A schematic view of EMLP (*left*) and a postoperative endoscopic view of a widely patent common frontal aperture (*right*).

from the field to maximize visualization but also to limit the transmission of heat to adjacent vital structures such as the optic apparatus and brain.

Drills have also influenced endosopic surgery of the orbit and lacrimal system. Endoscopic orbital techniques offer the advantages of enhanced visualization and more direct access to the posterior orbit and apex while also avoiding any facial scars. Performing a successful endoscopic dacryocystorhinostomy (E-DCR) for nasolacrimal duct obstruction requires the creation of a generous bony rhinostomy through, in part, the thick ascending process of the maxilla, with bone removal beginning in the region of the maxillary line and proceeding anteriorly.[10] Although many techniques for bone removal have been described, including the use of a mallet and osteotome, microdebriders, and lasers,[11–13] many surgeons prefer the finesse and precision best afforded by a high-speed drill.[10] Removal of thick bone during orbital decompression (for lateral and inferior walls especially) and optic nerve decompressions may also be augmented by the use of a drill.

The bone of the maxilla can also be removed posteriorly with a drill for exposure of the pterygopalatine fossa, as part of the endoscopic transpterygoid approach to the lateral recess of the sphenoid sinus.[14] Drills have also been applied for the transnasal resection of sinonasal fibro-osseous lesions[15] and large septal spurs during septoplasty.[16] The use of a drill is also recommended to superficially shave the underlying bone in cases of inverted papilloma to eliminate any small foci of tumor at the site of attachment. Even where the attachment is along the thin lamina papyracea, a diamond burr can be used to gain an added element of control after gross tumor has been removed.[17]

COBLATION
Technology

Coblation is a relatively new technology that was patented by ArthroCare (Austin, TX) in 1997, initially intended for cartilage ablation during arthroscopy. The Food and Drug Administration approved this technology for use in otolaryngology in 2000. It uses radiofrequency energy to energize electrolytes within a conductive medium (typically saline). This theoretically creates a plasma field that disrupts molecular bonds within the surrounding tissues at relatively low temperatures ($40°C-70°C$ as compared with more than $400°C$ with monopolar electrocautery). Because some studies suggest that a plasma field is unlikely to be created outside a vacuum, Zinder[18] theorized that the decreased thermal damage during coblation has more to do with vaporization of the saline solution than creation of a plasma field. In any event, there indeed does appear to be significantly less penetration of thermal energy into the surrounding tissue with the use of this technology, which may be advantageous.

Clinical Applications

The most common use of coblation in otolaryngology at the present time is during tonsillectomy, where some studies have suggested less postoperative pain and a faster recovery.[19] However, coblation is rapidly gaining popularity in rhinologic surgery for inferior turbinate reduction. Separate wands are available for adult and pediatric patients. Coblation is performed at several marked depths to create a series of ablated pockets submucosally within the erectile tissue of the inferior turbinate, which provides immediate volume reduction and will further scar down during healing (**Fig. 3**). Back and colleagues[20] showed significant subjective improvement in nasal obstruction, sneezing, crusting, and nasal discharge using a visual analog scale after coblation-mediated inferior turbinate reduction.[20] There is a paucity of well-designed

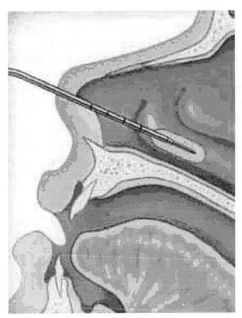

Fig. 3. Approach to coblation for inferior turbinate reduction. (*Courtesy of* ArthroCare, Austin, TX; with permission.)

randomized studies directly comparing coblation to other methods of turbinate reduction, but current literature does suggest promising short-term and even long-term results with this technique. Coblation has also been proposed for use in nasal polypectomy and transnasal tumor resection, where its hemostatic ability could provide essentially bloodless removal of soft tissue. However, there is little in the literature at the present time on this application. A major limitation to the use of currently available coblation technology to endoscopic sinus surgery for chronic sinusitis with or without nasal polyps is its inability to address the bony partitions encountered in the ethmoid sinus.

ULTRASONIC ASPIRATOR

One of the latest additions to the rhinologist's armamentarium is the bone-cutting ultrasonic aspirator, such as the CUSA NXT (Integra, Plainsboro, NJ). Ultrasonic aspirators operate on the converse piezoelectric effect, whereby application of an electric charge to certain crystals creates a reversible mechanical deformation (direct piezoelectric effect refers to electricity being generated by mechanical stress on the crystals). The piezoelectric effect was first described by Pierre and Jacques Curie in the late nineteenth century. Phacoemulsification techniques were originally used in cataract surgery, and ultrasonic instruments have since been developed for a wide variety of surgical specialties, including otolaryngology, where they were frequently used for cavitation of tumors including acoustic neuromas. Advances in ultrasonic technology now permit aspirators to expeditiously remove bone while still being respectful of nearby soft tissues.

Within the hand piece, a stack of piezoelectric discs or tubular piezoelectric crystal expands when exposed to positive voltage and contracts when the polarity is reversed, causing the attached bit to vibrate against the targeted tissue. This high-frequency vibration breaks down hydrogen bonds in tissue proteins, resulting in their denaturation. Cutting of tissue is secondary to cavitation, which is the formation, expansion, and subsequent implosion of small vapor bubbles within the tissue, caused by the ultrasonic waves. The resulting emulsified tissue is removed by continuous irrigation and suction. Constant suction (which can be adjusted by the surgeon) also helps pull more (soft) tissue against the tip to assist with tissue cavitation. The frequency of vibration can be optimized for either bone or soft tissue removal, giving it the advantage of tissue selectivity. Soft tissue aspirators tend to use a tubular tip with a longitudinal motion to cut tissue on the downstroke and emulsify it through cavitation on the upstroke. Newly designed bone-cutting aspirators tend to work along more conventional lines, with a grinding mechanism provided by longitudinal movement, torsional movement, or a combination of both, which emulsifies firm tissue such as bone. The ultrasonic aspirator reportedly generates less heat compared with conventional drills.

Technology

Ultrasonic aspirator systems are composed of a console that controls suction, irrigation, and power; two footpedals (one to engage the system, the other for pulsed irrigation); a hand piece with attached tip; and suction tubing. Suction and irrigation are applied to the back end of the hand piece, which also receives an electrical supply. The rate of suction and saline irrigation can be separately controlled to allow the surgeon to optimize the settings for a variety of tasks. The suction port is conveniently

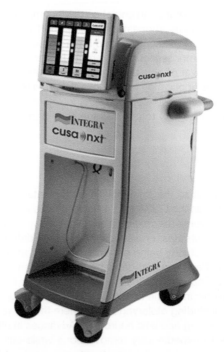

Fig. 4. The console of the CUSA NXT. This ultrasonic aspirator system functions on a digital technology platform that provides continuous feedback from the tip. (*Courtesy of* Integra, Plainsboro, NJ; with permission.)

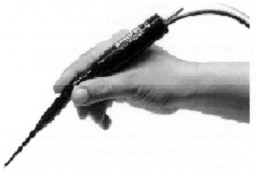

Fig. 5. The angled hand piece of an ultrasonic aspirator (Sonopet Omni). (*Courtesy of* Synergetics Inc, O'Fallon, MO; with permission.)

located at the distal aspect of the tip. Models are available from 23 to 36 kHz, all of which vibrate within a 0.36-mm range or less. CUSA NXT offers hand pieces that operate at 24 and 35 kHz, with the higher frequencies having a more focused and superficial tissue effect at the expense of power (making them best suited for detailed work around vital structures).

Power can be adjusted on the ultrasonic aspirator, with greater power resulting in increased amplitude of tip stroke and more aggressive takedown of bone or soft tissue. The CUSA NXT (**Fig. 4**) offers the advantage of a digital technology platform that provides continuous feedback depending on working conditions at the tip. Power is increased automatically when the tip is against tissue to maintain a steady frequency of vibration despite the added resistance. This allows the vibration frequency to be altered automatically and, in real time, to achieve pure sine wave resonance and to minimize harmonics, which results in improved efficiency.

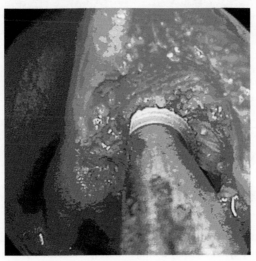

Fig. 6. Endoscopic view of an ultrasonic aspirator tip being used to create a large bony rhinostomy transnasally into the lacrimal fossa during E-DCR surgery for nasolacrimal duct obstruction.

The Sonopet Omni (Synergetics Inc, O'Fallon, MO) was developed in 1993, and it offers similar functioning and components as the CUSA NXT. The hand pieces have a slim profile to allow for easy passage into the nostrils, and they are angled to improve visualization of the working tip during surgery (**Fig. 5**). Design modifications (in hand pieces and tips) that would make these instruments more effective and ergonomic for transnasal endoscopic surgery are required.

Clinical Applications

The key advantage of the bone-cutting ultrasonic aspirator is that because it vibrates rather than spin like a drill burr or microdebrider blade, it is relatively atraumatic to the surrounding soft tissue and will not catch loose strips of mucosa or cotton pledgets. The lack of a spinning burr also reduces the risk of skipping or chatter associated with a conventional drill, providing more controlled takedown of thick bone. The use of

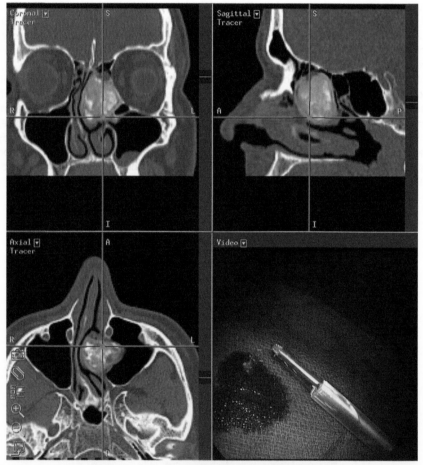

Fig. 7. Image-guidance system display during endoscopic resection of a large ethmoid fibro-osseous lesion attached to the lamina papyracea and skull base. Due to the tissue selectivity of this technology, the lesion was successfully resected without orbital or skull base injury using the ultrasonic aspirator (CUSA NXT tip shown in lower right panel).

bone-cutting ultrasonic aspirators has been described in a variety of neurosurgical procedures, and they have been praised for their ability to minimize damage to soft tissue structures (eg, vasculature and dura) while removing thick bone in confined spaces.[21]

The endoscopic use of these instruments was first described in otolaryngology by Antisdel and colleagues,[21] who reported their experience using the ultrasonic aspirator for the creation of the bony rhinostomy (**Fig. 6**) in E-DCR surgery.[21] The authors noted that inadvertent or even purposeful contact with the back of the vibrating tip of the aspirator with a mucosa-lined structure (such as the nasal septum or middle turbinate) did not cause any identifiable injury. Subsequently, a case report from the University of Pavia, Italy, described the use of the ultrasonic aspirator to successfully remove a frontoethmoidal osteoma transnasally.[22] The ability of this technology to selectively remove bone while being respectful of nearby mucosa and soft tissue holds considerable promise for minimizing adjacent trauma during endoscopic transnasal surgical procedures requiring significant bony removal (**Fig. 7**). The use of the surgical aspirator will likely increase as endoscopic sinus and neurorhinologic techniques continue to expand.

SUMMARY

Since the introduction of the microdebrider in the early 1990s, several other innovative powered tools, such as the endoscopic drill, coblator, and the ultrasonic aspirator, have been used during endoscopic sinus and skull base surgery. The primary drawback of powered instruments over conventional instrumentation continues to be the higher costs associated with their use, which include the initial capital expenditure for the system and ongoing costs of disposables (blades, bits, tips, and tubing). The main advantage is the ability to accomplish multiple functions, such as bone removal, suction, and irrigation, with one instrument. The effective use of any powered instrument requires an intimate understanding of its functioning, capabilities, and limitations.

REFERENCES

1. Kennedy DW, Kennedy EM. Endoscopic sinus surgery. AORN J 1985;42(6): 932–6.
2. Metson R, Sindwani R. Frontal sinusitis: endoscopic approaches. Otolaryngol Clin North Am 2004;37:411–22.
3. Draf W. Endonasal micro-endoscopic frontal sinus surgery: the Fulda concept. Oper Tech Oto Head Neck Surg 1991;2:234–40.
4. Gross WE, Gross CW, Becker D, et al. Modified transnasal endoscopic Lothrop procedure as an alternative to frontal sinus obliteration. Otolaryngol Head Neck Surg 1995;113:427–34.
5. Close LG, Lee NK, Leach JL, et al. Endoscopic resection of the intranasal frontal sinus floor. Ann Otol Rhinol Laryngol 1994;103:952–8.
6. Anderson P, Sindwani R. Safety and efficacy of the endoscopic modified Lothrop procedure: a systematic review and meta-analysis. Laryngoscope 2009;119(9): 1828–33.
7. Jho HD, Ha HG. Endoscopic endonasal skull base surgery: Part 1-The midline anterior fossa skull base. Minim Invasive Neurosurg 2004;47(1):1–8.
8. Jho HD, Ha HG. Endoscopic endonasal skull base surgery: Part 2-The cavernous sinus. Minim Invasive Neurosurg 2004;47(1):9–15.
9. Jho HD, Ha HG. Endoscopic endonasal skull base surgery: Part 3-The clivus and posterior fossa. Minim Invasive Neurosurg 2004;47(1):16–23.

10. Woog JJ, Sindwani R. Endoscopic dacryocystorhinostomy and conjunctivoda-cryocystorhinostomy. Otolaryngol Clin North Am 2006;39(5):1001–17.
11. Cokkeser Y, Evereklioglu C, Tercan M, et al. Hammer-chisel technique in endo-scopic dacryocystorhinostomy. Ann Otol Rhinol Laryngol 2003;112(5):444–9.
12. Yoon SW, Yoon YS, Lee SH. Clinical results of endoscopic dacryocystorhinostomy using a microdebrider. Korean J Ophthalmol 2006;20(1):1–6.
13. Maini S, Raghava N, Youngs R, et al. Endoscopic endonasal laser versus endo-nasal surgical dacryocystorhinostomy for epiphora due to nasolacrimal duct obstruction: prospective, randomised, controlled trial. J Laryngol Otol 2007; 121(12):1170–6. Epub 2007 Jun 29.
14. Bolger WE. Endoscopic transpterygoid approach to the lateral sphenoid recess: surgical approach and clinical experience. Otolaryngol Head Neck Surg 2005; 133(1):20–6.
15. Samaha M, Metson R. Image-guided resection of fibro-osseous lesions of the skull base. Am J Rhinol 2003;17(2):115–8.
16. Giles WC, Gross CW, Gross WE, et al. Endoscopic septoplasty. Laryngoscope 1994;104:1507–9.
17. Chandra RK, Schlosser R, Kennedy DW. Use of the 70-degree diamond burr in the management of complicated frontal sinus disease. Laryngoscope 2004; 114(2):188–92.
18. Zinder DJ. Common myths about electrosurgery. Otolaryngol Head Neck Surg 2000;123:450–5.
19. Magdy EA, Elwany S, el-Daly AS, et al. Coblation tonsillectomy: a prospective, double-blind, randomised, clinical and histopathological comparison with dissec-tion-ligation, monopolar electrocautery and laser tonsillectomies. J Laryngol Otol 2008;122(3):282–90. Epub 2007 Nov 26.
20. Back LJ, Hytonen ML, Malmberg HO, et al. Submucosal bipolar radiofrequency thermal ablation of inferior turbinates: a long-term follow-up with subjective and objective assessment. Laryngoscope 2002;112:1806–12.
21. Antisdel JL, Kadze MS, Sindwani R. Application of ultrasonic aspirator to endo-scopic dacrocystorhinostomy. Otolaryngol Head Neck Surg 2008;139(4):586–8.
22. Pagella F, Giourgos G, Matti E, et al. Removal of a fronto-ethmoidal osteoma using the Sonopet Omni bone curette: first impressions. Laryngoscope 2008; 118(2):307–9.

Advances in Surgical Navigation

Dary J. Costa, MD, Raj Sindwani, MD, FACS, FRCS(C)*

KEYWORDS

- Image guidance • Surgical navigation
- Computer-assisted surgery • Endoscopic sinus surgery
- Frameless stereotaxy • Image fusion

Endoscopic sinus surgery using rigid endoscopes is now the conventional technique for opening obstructed and diseased sinus outflow tracts. Although the application of endoscopes has revolutionized the diagnosis and surgical management of sinonasal disorders, a major limitation continues to be that the view is not in three dimensions. When operating from only a two-dimensional magnified image, localization of instruments within the sinonasal cavity during surgery depends largely upon the depth of penetration and the quality of tactile feedback. Additionally, surgical orientation may be limited by distorted anatomy, extensive polyposis, or intraoperative bleeding. Navigation technology may be viewed as a method to improve visualization during surgery and serves as an adjunct to nasal endoscopy. Surgical navigation systems can be employed to determine the precise location of critical structures during the course of an operation.

Navigation systems identify anatomic landmarks by locating surgical instruments in space, calculating the location of the instrument tip in relation to the patient, and projecting the instrument location onto a previously obtained imaging study (usually computed tomography [CT]). The operator can use this information for intraoperative surgical navigation or preoperative planning using the computer workstation, which displays the patient's images simultaneously in all three anatomic planes (coronal, axial, and sagittal).

SURGICAL NAVIGATION COMPONENTS
Imaging Data

CT scans are the imaging modality of choice when evaluating the paranasal sinuses and are used routinely for image-guided surgery. The detailed bony anatomy provided by high-resolution CT imaging accentuates the surgical landmarks and the confines of the sinonasal cavity. The unit of data in CT imaging is cuboidal and permits reconstruction of images in the coronal, axial, or sagittal plane. Thinner slices improve

Department of Otolaryngology—Head & Neck Surgery, St Louis University School of Medicine, 6th Floor FDT, 3635 Vista Ave at Grand Blvd, St Louis, MO 63110, USA
* Corresponding author.
E-mail address: sindwani@slu.edu (R. Sindwani).

Otolaryngol Clin N Am 42 (2009) 799–811
doi:10.1016/j.otc.2009.07.004
0030-6665/09/$ – see front matter © 2009 Published by Elsevier Inc.

resolution. The optimal CT scan is an axial CT with 1-mm slice thickness and a 512 × 512-pixel matrix.[1]

Magnetic Resonance Imaging (MRI) provides excellent soft tissue detail and is frequently incorporated into image-guidance systems for intracranial procedures. MRI is also extremely useful in the evaluation of sinonasal conditions, such as allergic fungal sinusitis and neoplasia, precisely detailing the site and extension of benign and malignant sinonasal tumors. MRI is also useful in evaluating encephaloceles and cerebrospinal fluid leaks, as the high-intensity signal of cerebrospinal fluid in the sinuses on T2-weighted imaging can suggest the presence of a leak. Like CT data, MRI data can be loaded into an image-guidance system and used for intraoperative navigation.

Traditionally, the imaging data are obtained preoperatively and transferred to the image-guidance system computer through digital storage media, such as universal serial bus (USB) sticks or compact disk–read-only memory (CD-ROM) disks. Newer systems have the capacity to directly download data via high-speed Internet or wireless Ethernet connections, making data transfer from radiology to the navigation system in the operating room simple and seamless.[2] Until recently, most available image-guidance systems required a special proprietary CT protocol for the data set to be incorporated into the software and CT scans performed elsewhere (referred to as *foreign* data sets) were not usable for navigation. This was a major shortcoming, as it mandated repeat imaging, thus exposing the patient to further radiation, adding to inconvenience, and increasing cost, solely for the purpose of employing navigation. Manufacturers of most systems have resolved this issue such that the majority of foreign data sets available in electronic format are now suitable for navigation provided they conform to a few common parameters. These vary somewhat by manufacturer but frequently include axial cuts with a 512×512-pixel matrix, 3-mm or less slice thickness, and a 0° gantry tilt.[3] This has been a significant improvement in software design for these systems, and has made navigation easier to use.

Registration

Registration is the establishment of a rigid relationship between two coordinate systems: (1) the images previously obtained and (2) an arbitrary system employed to describe every point within the surgical field. After registration is performed, a navigation system is capable of translating from any point on the patient to the same point on the imaging study using a transformation matrix.

Three types of registration are currently available: paired-point registration, automatic registration, and contour-based registration.[4] The paired-point method requires the surgeon to designate fiducial points on both the patient and imaging data. Accuracy can be improved by increasing the number of points and using a distribution of fiducial points to encompass the three-dimensional area of surgical interest. A greater number of paired points is desirable; however, a greater number of points increases the time for registration and does not significantly improve accuracy. Most surgeons recommend 6 to 10 paired points in a nonlinear distribution around the surgical area.[4] Automatic registration requires a headset that is placed on the patient at the time of CT or MRI. The headset, embedded with metal fiducials, is designed to fit the patient in a reproducible fashion and it must be reapplied and worn during surgery. The image-guidance system recognizes points within the headset and uses these for "automatic" registration. The accuracy of this method depends on consistent placement of the headset. Contour-based registration requires the image-guidance system to build a three-dimensional model of surface contours of the patient's face using the imaging data. A standard probe or reflected laser light can then be used to define the surface contour of the patient at the time of surgery. This technique rapidly defines a large number of registration points (40–500). The contour method loses accuracy if the patient's surface contour changes from the time of image collection to the time of surgery because of edema, weight gain, and stretching from surgical drapes. Early registration paradigms were difficult to follow,[5] but recent features, such as touch screens, auto-registration, and surface registration, have simplified the process significantly. Most systems now employ either automatic or surface registration given the greater simplicity of these techniques. Multiple clinical trials have shown all three registration systems to be reliable with accuracies of 1 to 2 mm.[6,7]

Tracking Technology

Tracking is a method of dynamically following the movement of an instrument in space, calculating the location of the instrument in relation to the patient, and projecting the location of the instrument onto an imaging study. The two tracking systems currently available are optical- and electromagnetic-based systems. Both systems are highly accurate to within a few millimeters and both systems account for intraoperative head position by fastening a headset to the patient.

Electromagnetic systems track instruments using a radiofrequency transmitter within a special headset and a receiver positioned within the instrument. The headset, containing embedded fiducial markers, and trackable instruments are attached via wires to the system hardware. The headset must be worn during the preoperative CT scan and again intraoperatively. Electromagnetic tracking may be susceptible to interference from metal instruments within the field or the metal operating room table. Thus, metal devices and anesthesia equipment must be placed an appropriate distance away from the operating field and some investigators recommend placing extra padding between the patient and the table.[8]

Optical systems use infrared light and a camera positioned 6 ft (approximately 1.8 m) above the patient's head to track instruments (**Fig. 1**). This provides a wireless mechanism for instrument localization, but requires a clear pathway between the tracking device and the instruments. Equipment and draping must be placed carefully to avoid line-of-sight obstruction.

Specialized equipment and instruments are needed for both types of systems. Optical tracking systems require light-reflecting spheres (also referred to as *stars* or *glions*) attached to the proximal end of wireless surgical instruments. Electromagnetic

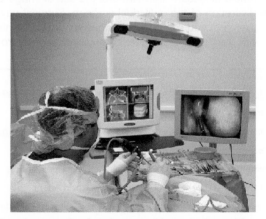

Fig. 1. Intraoperative photograph of an image-guidance system with an infrared tracking camera.

platforms require the attachment of a wired probe to the instruments. Both systems allow for a variety of instruments to be tracked, including probes, straight and angled suctions, and curettes. With the optical-based systems, however, a recent innovation known as *universal calibration* allows reflective spheres to be affixed to any rigid instrument, thus permitting navigation with any surgical instrument including drills and microdebriders. The computer workstation integrates the data set with information from the tracking system and projects the location of the instrument tip.[9]

During the course of surgery, the surgeon must frequently corroborate the accuracy of the image-guidance system using obvious surface and intranasal landmarks, such as the tip of the nose or the posterior wall of the maxillary sinus. A change in the angle of the instrument facing an optical tracking device or movement of the headset can change the projected location and contribute to inaccuracies and drift.[6]

SURGICAL NAVIGATION INDICATIONS

In general, the indications for surgical navigation are situations in which additional information beyond the endoscopic or surgical view is beneficial. This includes situations involving patients with advanced disease or unusual pathology.[10] Patients undergoing intervention for disease in close proximity to critical structures, such as the skull base or orbit, or in cases where the disease extends to difficult-to-reach anatomic locations (perhaps even beyond the paranasal sinuses) would benefit from surgical navigation. The American Academy of Otolaryngology has endorsed the use of image-guidance and has described examples of indications for navigation (**Box 1**).[11] In addition to the intraoperative advantage with image-guidance, the display of the imaging data in three simultaneous planes can be a very powerful tool for preoperative planning, particularly important in more complex cases. Surgical navigation may also improve resident training by demonstrating anatomic relationships and allowing for monitoring of resident progress.[12]

Surgical navigation is helpful, but not necessary, in patients with intermediate disease. Examples include patients with obstruction of the frontal or sphenoid outflow tract. However, an image-guidance system can be invaluable for procedures, involving revision surgery on the frontal and sphenoid sinuses.

Surgical navigation is not necessary in patients with disease localized to the maxillary and anterior ethmoid sinuses.[10] Furthermore, the use of image-guidance should be left to the sole discretion of the individual surgeon. Surgical navigation may not be needed for any given procedure if the experienced surgeon is comfortable performing the operation with traditional techniques. Many endoscopic procedures can be

---

Box 1
American Academy of Otolaryngology—Head & Neck Surgery indications for image-guided surgery

o Revision sinus surgery

o Distorted sinus anatomy of development, postoperative, or traumatic origin

o Extensive sinonasal polyposis

o Pathology involving the frontal, posterior ethmoid, and sphenoid sinuses

o Disease abutting the skull base, orbit, optic nerve, or carotid artery

o Cerebrospinal fluid rhinorrhea or conditions where there is a skull-base defect

o Benign and malignant sinonasal neoplasms

performed safely with standard equipment. Therefore, use of image guidance is not standard of care.

EXPANDED APPLICATIONS

Recently, external approaches to the sinuses have also been augmented through the use of surgical navigation. Frontal sinus obliteration via the osteoplastic flap technique is a prime example. Traditionally, a radiographic template has been used to guide osteotomies through the frontal bone around the perimeter of the frontal sinus to expose the sinus interior. A high rate of complications has been encountered as a result of misdirected osteotomies. These complications include inadvertent orbital or intracranial penetration.[13] Previous commercially available systems required a standard headset that obstructs access to the forehead area. Through the use of a skull fixation array positioned in an unobtrusive location away from the forehead, the need for a standard headset is obviated, and an image-guidance system can be used to accurately demarcate the perimeter of the frontal sinus once the frontal bone is exposed. The application of an image-guidance system to osteoplastic flap–approach frontal sinus obliteration has been shown to reduce intraoperative complications.[14]

Surgical navigation is extremely useful in skull-base surgery. Navigation can assist in ensuring adequate resection of tumors and help determine the extent of inflammatory diseases involving the skull base. Petrous apex lesions can be approached via transsphenoidal or transpalatine approaches[15] and image-guidance can be used to identify and preserve the carotid artery or cavernous sinus. Image-guidance systems are ideally suited to bony tumors, but also aid in the endoscopic resection of soft tissue tumors by assisting in defining boundaries for resection (bony skull base) and avoiding adjacent vital structures.[16] Transsphenoidal resection of pituitary tumors and other transsphenoidal procedures have been greatly facilitated by the application of image-guidance.[17] Endoscopic management of encephaloceles and cerebrospinal fluid rhinorrhea is augmented by surgical navigation as well (**Fig. 2**).

Endoscopic orbital procedures, such as dacryocystorhinostomy, orbital decompression, and optic nerve decompression, may also be enhanced with image-guidance. During orbital and optic nerve decompression, key landmarks in the area of the orbital apex, including the lateral sphenoid face, sphenoethmoid angle, and opticocarotid recess, can be identified with near certainty.[18] In addition, the preoperative image-guidance evaluation helps identify the association between the sphenoid architecture, optic canal, and the proximity of the carotid artery. Variants, such as sphenoethmoid cells (Onodi cells), with possible dehiscence of either the carotid artery or optic nerve are better characterized by the three-plane images of an image-guidance system. Removal of optic canal bone can be done with greater confidence with simultaneous visualization of the carotid path and intracranial border.[18]

Surgical navigation systems have also influenced pediatric sinonasal surgery. The definition of pediatric sinusitis and the surgical approaches used have been evolving over the last decade. Certain sinus conditions found in the pediatric population are especially amenable to the use of intraoperative navigation. Examples include the extensive polyposis of cystic fibrosis, allergic fungal sinusitis, and endoscopic choanal atresia repair (**Fig. 3**). Recent reports demonstrate efficacy of image guidance for periorbital abscesses and juvenile nasopharyngeal angiofibroma.[19,20] The authors of a recent review concluded that image guidance was indicated for advanced sinonasal procedures in children.[21]

Finally, the use of surgical navigation appears to be expanding to non-sinonasal otolaryngologic applications as well. A report has been published on the use of

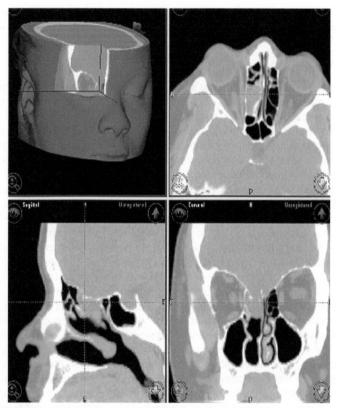

Fig. 2. Screen shot of an encephalocele projected in the coronal, axial, and sagittal plane on an image-guidance system.

surgical navigation to identify retropharyngeal lymph nodes in a patient with metastatic carcinoma.[22]

EFFICACY AND IMPACT ON OUTCOMES

A recent survey demonstrated that 73% of otolaryngologists use image-guidance with over 80% of respondents agreeing that it provides safer surgery.[23] However, the low complication rate encountered in routine endoscopic sinus surgery would require a very large scale effort to definitively demonstrate that navigation systems reduce complications in endoscopic sinus surgery. Additionally, randomized controlled studies on the efficacy and outcomes of image guidance are difficult to conduct for ethical reasons.[24] Several investigators have suggested that the complication rate of sinus surgery may be reduced by employing surgical navigation technology. Fried and colleagues[25] performed a retrospective review comparing sinonasal procedures on patients before image-guidance systems were available with current procedures and concluded that image-guidance may reduce complications. Tabaee and colleagues[26] studied 85 patients who underwent revision surgery with surgical navigation and reported no serious complications within this group. These results can be compared with data published by Jiang and Hsu,[27] who reported a 9.9% complication rate in cases of revision endoscopic sinus surgery without image-guidance. However, the data presented by Jiang and Hsu were obtained from 1988 to 1998 and there are

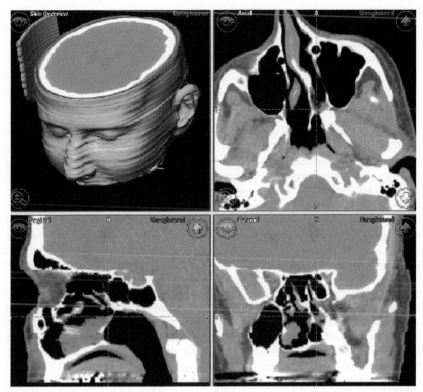

Fig. 3. Image-guidance system being used to confirm the location of a unilateral choanal atresia.

likely to have been other improvements in revision endoscopic sinus surgery since that review. Sindwani and Metson[14] demonstrated a significant decrease in complications when using surgical navigation for frontal sinus localization during the osteoplastic flap obliteration procedure when compared with traditional non–image guidance methods. Studies by Metson[28] and Tabaee,[29] however, found no significant difference in complication rates between routine endoscopic sinus surgery performed with and without surgical navigation.

The use of surgical navigation may influence patient outcome. In a review of 800 sinus procedures done at a community hospital, Reardon noted a significant increase in the number of frontal sinuses entered after the introduction of image-guidance.[30] Success rates for complex procedures, such as frontal drill-out surgery with and without image-guidance, are statistically comparable, although there appears to be a trend toward higher surgical success rates when the image-guidance system is employed.[31] Surgical navigation is a valuable adjunct in the endoscopic management of cerebrospinal fluid rhinorrhea but image-guidance does not statistically improve rates of successful closure.[32] Dubin and colleagues[33] studied the use of image-guidance in orbital decompression and did not identify a statistically significant difference in outcomes or complications using this technology.

Perioperative quality of life has been compared with and without surgical navigation. Javer and Genoway[34] demonstrated a greater overall improvement in quality of life in patients undergoing sinus surgery performed with an image-guidance system. However, Tabaee and colleagues[29] concluded that image-guidance does not affect quality-of-life outcomes in patients undergoing sinus surgery for chronic sinusitis.

There is a steep learning curve when using new technology. Surgeons should start with relatively easy cases when learning to use an image-guidance system. Initially using image guidance for routine procedures establishes familiarity with the equipment so that the surgeon will feel comfortable using the system on more challenging cases.

LIMITATIONS OF SURGICAL NAVIGATION

The "costs" of surgical navigation include the cost of increased time expenditure, the cost of disruption in the "flow" of the operation, and financial cost.[35] Metson and colleagues[28] demonstrated an average increase in operative time of 17.4 min/case, commenting that this will likely improve as the learning curve associated with this new technology plateaus over time. Based on operating-room and anesthesia charges, this increase in time resulted in an additional charge of approximately $500 per case. However, selection bias may account for some of these findings as operations involving surgical navigation are usually more complex and therefore possibly of longer duration. It is also possible that as a result of the application of image guidance, the surgeon could improve efficiency and reduce complications, which may actually decrease the operative length. Another consideration is that image-guidance systems have become much more user-friendly as software and computing power have evolved. This has shortened set-up times and reduced lengthy trouble-shooting episodes. Revenues captured from the use of *Current Procedural Terminology* code 61795 for image-guidance systems (stereotactic computer-assisted volumetric navigation procedure) although variable, must also factor into the financial analysis when the decision to purchase a system is entertained.

The main expense for using surgical navigation is the initial capital expenditure for the device. Several companies now offer economical compact ("basic") units promoted for the ambulatory surgery center market for about half of the cost of larger units with advanced features. Through the development of these smaller and less-expensive models, the industry has responded to the growing trend of performing outpatient endoscopic sinus surgery in ambulatory surgery centers, thus altering the landscape of image-guided surgery such that navigational technology is no longer limited to large academic centers.

Surgical navigation systems will only work as well as the quality of imaging study supplied. A CT scan with 3-mm slices will have an accuracy of only 3 mm at best, even when registration is 100% accurate. Additionally, it is important to have the entire skin surface captured within the study as the registration process involves the surface of the patient's face. Patient headsets worn intraoperatively allow for real-time tracking but are prone to movement while the patient is manipulated, thus decreasing accuracy and introducing drift. Frequent corroboration with the clinical landmarks and evaluation of the headset for possible movement during a case will allow such movement to be identified and addressed early. For the optical-based systems, maintaining a clear line of sight from the camera to the instruments can be challenging, especially during complex procedures where the endoscope may block the reflective spheres on the instruments or if the instruments are being used at unconventional angles. Although unbound from issues related to line of sight, electromagnetic systems have their own limitations, including problems with cords looping over the surgical field and interference from nearby metal objects.

Finally, although navigation systems are highly accurate, they are also fallible. These systems are simply an adjunct to clinical expertise and experience. When information from the image-guidance system conflicts with clinical judgment, trust your judgment.

FUTURE MODIFICATIONS

A new market has emerged for stations that are more compact and portable, potentially even allowing for transport between ambulatory surgery centers or for servicing more remote rural communities. As ambulatory surgery centers become more popular, they will provide significant market pressure for smaller and even cheaper navigation systems (**Fig. 4**). In the foreseeable future, all of the hardware components of image-guidance systems will become integrated into the endoscopic operating room suite, and will become invisible to the surgeon. Incorporation of robotic technology and voice-activated controls for image-guidance systems also seems likely.

Universal instrument registration (calibration), at least for optical-based systems, has expanded the range of instruments that can be used for navigation, such that almost any rigid instrument can be tracked. The electromagnetic system, due to its platform, is not currently as amenable to such variations because it requires hard (wired) instrument connections. The next revolutionary innovation in navigation will be the ability to track flexible instruments, such as catheter tips placed deep within body cavities or structures. Such an innovation will certainly rely on an electromagnetic platform (providing liberation from line-of-sight concerns) and will have a far-reaching impact in the medical field beyond just our specialty. Software advances will also allow for more complex three-dimensional modeling of patient anatomy for

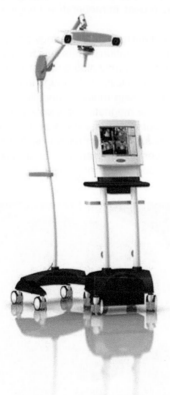

Fig. 4. Example of a compact image-guidance system (Kolibri; BrainLAB, AG, Munich, Germany). Compact, economical systems are well suited to ambulatory surgical centers. (*From* BrainLAB, AG, Munich, Germany; with permission.)

preoperative surgical planning. Options and indications for multimodal navigation will undoubtedly grow.

A central concern of surgeons using image-guidance is that navigation is based upon static preoperative images that do not reflect intraoperative changes. This is not a major issue during the majority of endoscopic sinus surgery procedures for inflammatory disease because the bony peripheral boundaries of the sinonasal tract (skull base, septum, and orbit) are left undisturbed. However, as more complex pathology and expanded approaches evolve, navigating from static data will become a limiting issue. Effective intraoperative imaging with data-set updates likely represents the next major step in the evolution of image-guidance technology.[36] Intraoperative MRI is currently being used in selected neurosurgical procedures in some centers and has been described for endoscopic sinus surgery.[37] Intraoperative CT scanning can be performed quickly, successfully, and has led to a change in the surgical plan in up to 30% of patients.[38] Recent attempts for intraoperative updates have also been performed using fluoroscopy (as a more practical proxy for CT image data).[39] However, real-time imaging complicates the operation by adding time and increasing costs significantly. In addition, intraoperative imaging is almost invariably inferior to images obtained with scanners designed purely for diagnosis.[40] Finally, intraoperative bleeding may be misinterpreted as soft tissue and lead to misdirected surgery. As portable CT imaging systems become smaller, faster, and less expensive, repeat intraoperative imaging is sure to find its way into the operating theater.

Recent advances in surgical navigation technology permit the surgeon to navigate using CT images, MRIs, or a combination of data sets fused together or superimposed (**Fig. 5**).[41] Other imaging modalities may also be incorporated to provide even more information to further enhance localization. Although infrequently encountered, there are situations where navigation using multiple modalities may prove advantageous, such as using CT angiography or magnetic resonance angiography during extended intracranial/skull-base procedures for lesions near the internal carotid or basilar arteries.[42] Emerging modalities, such as positron emission tomography scanning, which study functional changes rather than structural abnormalities, may also one day become useful to endoscopic surgeons as well.[43]

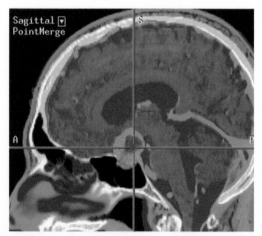

Fig. 5. Fusion image with bone landmarks from a CT study and the soft tissue detail of a pituitary tumor from a magnetic resonance study.

SUMMARY

Surgical navigation is safe, accurate, and holds considerable power for improving patient care. Available navigation systems continue to improve as evidenced by the current widespread use in endoscopic sinonasal surgery. This technology has established itself as a valuable adjunctive tool for the endoscopic surgeon. Indications for navigation continue to expand as imaging data synthesis evolves to include multimodality fusion and real-time intraoperative data-set updates. Technology is not a substitute for proper technique or experience, however, and the use of navigation for any given procedure is not presently standard of care.

REFERENCES

1. Aygun N, Zinreich SJ. Imaging for functional endoscopic sinus surgery. Otolaryngol Clin North Am 2006;39:403–16.
2. Fried MP, Parikh SR, Sadoughi B. Image-guidance for endoscopic sinus surgery. Laryngoscope 2008;118(7):1287–92.
3. Anon JB, Klimek L. Stereotactic surgery. In: Levine H, Clemente P, editors. Sinus surgery; endoscopic and microscopic approaches. New York: Theime Medical Publishers; 2005. p. 219–30.
4. Citardi M, Batra P. Image-guided sinus surgery: current concepts and technology. Otolaryngol Clin North Am 2005;38:439–52.
5. Metson R, Cosenza MJ, Cunningham MJ, et al. Physician experience with an optical image-guidance system for sinus surgery. Laryngoscope 2000;110: 972–6.
6. Fried MP, Kleefield J, Gopal H, et al. Image-guided endoscopic surgery: results of accuracy and performance in a multicenter clinical study using an electromagnetic tracking system. Laryngoscope 1997;107:594–601.
7. Anon JB. Computer-aided endoscopic sinus surgery. Laryngoscope 1998;108: 949–61.
8. Metson R, Gliklich RE, Cosenza M. A comparison of image-guidance systems for sinus surgery. Laryngoscope 1998;108:1164–70.
9. Reardon EJ. The impact of image-guidance systems on sinus surgery. Otolaryngol Clin North Am 2005;38:515–25.
10. Metson R, Gray S. Image-guided sinus surgery: practical considerations. Otolaryngol Clin North Am 2005;38:527–34.
11. AAO–HNS policy on intra-operative use of computer-aided surgery. American Academy of Otolaryngology—Head and Neck Surgery (AAO–HNS). Available at: http://www.entnet.org/Practice/policyIntraOperativeSurgery.cfm. Accessed May 10, 2009.
12. Casiano RR, Numa WA Jr. Efficacy of computed tomographic image–guided endoscopic sinus surgery in residency training programs. Laryngoscope 2000; 110:1277–82.
13. Weber R, Draf W, Keerl R, et al. Osteoplastic frontal sinus surgery with fat obliteration: technique and long-term results using magnetic resonance imaging in 82 operations. Laryngoscope 2000;110:1037–44.
14. Sindwani R, Metson R. Impact of image-guidance on complications during osteoplastic frontal sinus surgery. Otolaryngol Head Neck Surg 2004;131:150–5.
15. Zanation AM, Snyderman CH, Carrau RL, et al. Endoscopic endonasal surgery for petrous apex lesions. Laryngoscope 2009;119(1):19–25.
16. Schlosser R, Bolger W. Image-guided procedures of the skull base. Otolaryngol Clin North Am 2005;38:483–90.

17. Javer AR, Marglani O, Lee A, et al. Image-guided endoscopic transsphenoidal removal of pituitary tumours. J Otolaryngol Head Neck Surg 2008;37(4):474–80.
18. Pletcher S, Sindwani R, Metson R. Endoscopic orbital and optic nerve decompression. Otolaryngol Clin North Am 2006;39:943–58.
19. White JB, Parikh SR. Early experience with image guidance in endoscopic transnasal drainage of periorbital abscesses. J Otolaryngol 2005;34:63–5.
20. Mair EA, Battiata A, Casler JD. Endoscopic laser-assisted excision of juvenile nasopharyngeal angiofibromas. Arch Otolaryngol Head Neck Surg 2003;129:454–9.
21. Parikh SR, Cuellar H, Sadoughi B, et al. Indications for image-guidance in pediatric sinonasal surgery. Int J Pediatr Otorhinolaryngol 2009;73(3):351–6.
22. Mierzwa K, Mueller A. Image-guided surgery in an occult neck metastasis. Head Neck 2009. Available at: http://dx.doi.org/10.1002/hed.21118. Accessed May 10, 2009.
23. Hepworth EJ, Bucknor M, Patel A, et al. Nationwide survey on the use of image-guided functional endoscopic sinus surgery. Otolaryngol Head Neck Surg 2006; 135:73–5.
24. Smith TL, Stewart MG, Orlandi RR, et al. Indications for image-guided sinus surgery: the current evidence. Am J Rhinol 2007;21:80–3.
25. Fried MP, Moharir VM, Shin J, et al. Comparison of endoscopic sinus surgery with and without image guidance. Am J Rhinol 2002;16:193–7.
26. Tabaee A, Kacker A, Kassenoff TL, et al. Outcome of computer assisted sinus surgery; a 5-year study. Am J Rhinol 2003;17:291–7.
27. Jiang RS, Hsu CY. Revision functional endoscopic sinus surgery. Ann Otol Rhinol Laryngol 2002;111:155–9.
28. Metson R, Cosenza M, Gliklich RE, et al. The role of image-guidance systems for head and neck surgery. Arch Otolaryngol Head Neck Surg 1999;125:1100–4.
29. Tabaee A, Hsu AK, Shrime MG, et al. Quality of life and complications following image-guided endoscopic sinus surgery. Otolaryngol Head Neck Surg 2006; 135:76–80.
30. Reardon EJ. Navigational risks associated with sinus surgery and the clinical effects of implementing a navigational system for sinus surgery. Laryngoscope 2002;112:1–19.
31. Sindwani R, Metson R. Image-guided frontal sinus surgery. Otolaryngol Clin North Am 2005;38:461–71.
32. Tabaee A, Kassenoff TL, Kacker A, et al. The efficacy of computer assisted surgery in the endoscopic management of cerebrospinal fluid rhinorrhea. Otolaryngol Head Neck Surg 2005;133:936–43.
33. Dubin MR, Tabaee A, Scruggs JT, et al. Image-guided endoscopic orbital decompression for Graves' orbitopathy. Ann Otol Rhinol Laryngol 2008;117(3): 177–85.
34. Javer AR, Genoway KA. Patient quality of life improvements with and without computer assistance in sinus surgery: outcomes study. J Otolaryngol 2006; 35(6):373–9.
35. Hemmerdinger SA, Jacobs JB, Lebowitz RA. Accuracy and cost analysis of image-guided sinus surgery. Otolaryngol Clin North Am 2005;38:453–60.
36. Sindwani R, Bucholz RD. The next generation of navigational technology. Otolaryngol Clin North Am 2005;38:551–62.
37. Fried MP, Hsu L, Topulos GP, et al. Image-guided surgery in a new magnetic resonance suite: preclinical considerations. Laryngoscope 1996;106:411–7.
38. Jackman AH, Palmer JN, Chiu AG, et al. Use of intraoperative CT scanning in endoscopic sinus surgery: a preliminary report. Am J Rhinol 2008;22(2):170–4.

39. Brown SM, Sadoughi B, Cuellar H, et al. Feasibility of near real-time image-guided sinus surgery using intraoperative fluoroscopic computed axial tomography. Otolaryngol Head Neck Surg 2007;136:268–73.
40. Cartellieri M, Vorbeck F. Endoscopic sinus surgery using intraoperative computed tomography imaging for updating a three-dimensional navigation system. Laryngoscope 2000;110:292–6.
41. Leong JL, Batra PS, Citardi MJ. CT-MR image fusion for the management of skull base lesions. Otolaryngol Head Neck Surg 2006;134:868–76.
42. Leong JL, Batra PS, Citardi MJ. Three-dimensional computed tomography angiography of the internal carotid artery for preoperative evaluation of sinonasal lesions and intraoperative surgical navigation. Laryngoscope 2005;115:1618–23.
43. Pirotte BJ, Levivier M, Goldman S, et al. Positron emission tomography-guided volumetric resection of supratentorial high-grade gliomas: a survival analysis in 66 consecutive patients. Neurosurgery 2009;64(3):471–81.

Advances in Absorbable Biomaterials and Nasal Packing

Rowan Valentine, MBBS[a], Peter-John Wormald, MD[a],*,
Raj Sindwani, MD, FACS, FRCS(C)[b]

KEYWORDS

- Endoscopic sinus surgery • Biomaterials • Hemostasis
- Chronic rhinosinusitis • Adhesion

BACKGROUND: NASAL PACKING IN ENDOSCOPIC SINUS SURGERY

Endoscopic sinus surgery (ESS) is a continuously developing field that has had many exciting developments in the past 3 decades. Advances in the understanding of functional sinus surgery and mucosal-sparing techniques has driven an interest in the management of the post-ESS nasal and sinus cavity to achieve more rapid postoperative reepithelialization and reciliation. Many surgeons believe that the postoperative treatment regimen is as important as the surgery.

All sinus surgeons have the common objective of achieving excellent hemostasis and postoperative healing that avoids adhesion formation and lateralization of the middle turbinate; however, little agreement exists on how this is best achieved. The use of various interventions, from removable nasal packing, absorbable nasal packing, to no packing at all, is widely debated.

Nasal packing has been the traditional method of controlling ongoing bleeding after surgery to the paranasal sinuses. Additionally, nasal packing has been used to prevent adhesion formation, middle turbinate lateralization, and restenosis after surgery. Unfortunately, removable nasal packing has been rated by patients to be the most unpleasant aspect of the ESS surgical experience.[1,2] Some surgeons advocate not packing the middle meatus,[3] whereas others continue to use this technique to prevent middle turbinate lateralization.[4] Controversy still exists about whether to pack or not.

Disclosures and Conflict of interest: Dr Wormald is part of a consortium that has patented the use of chitosan gel in the nose. He receives royalties from Medtronic ENT for instruments designed and is a consultant for Neilmed Pharmaceuticals. Dr Sindwani received an educational grant from Medafor, Inc in 2007.

[a] Department of Surgery-Otorhinolaryngology, Head and Neck Surgery, The Queen Elizabeth Hospital, University of Adelaide, 28 Woodville Road, Woodville, Adelaide, SA 5011, Australia
[b] Department of Otolaryngology, St Louis University Hospital, 3635 Vista Avenue, St Louis, MO 63110, USA
* Corresponding author.
E-mail address: http://peterj.wormald@adelaide.edu.au (P-J. Wormald).

This article reviews the literature on the use of absorbable biomaterials and their effects on hemostasis and wound healing, evaluating experiences with 20th century agents and exploring developing trends and 21st century innovations.

Nasal packing was first described in the otorhinolaryngolic literature in 1951[5] and the use of absorbable biomaterials since 1969.[6] Removable nasal packing has been designed to tamponade mucosal bleeding and act as a barrier to adhesion formation. Numerous packing agents are available, including Vaseline-soaked ribbon gauze, fingerstall packs, polyvinyl acetate sponge (Merocel, Medtronic Xomed, Jacksonville, Florida), and various balloon tamponade devices. However, these agents cause considerable discomfort for patients, both in terms of pain and bleeding on removal.[1,2,7–9] Other complications associated with removable nasal packing include septal perforation, pack dislodgement, aspiration, toxic shock syndrome, foreign body granuloma, myospherulosis, obstructive sleep apnea secondary to nasal obstruction, and even death.[10,11] Animal studies investigating the mucosal trauma caused by removable nasal packing have shown a 50% to 70% loss of the ciliated mucosal surface area in the region of the pack.[12] Therefore, a transient impairment of the patient's innate immune system, the mucociliary clearance, may be associated with the use of removable nasal packing.[13]

These drawbacks of removable nasal packing have led to the ongoing development and application of absorbable biomaterials that do not require subsequent removal and still achieve positive effects on hemostasis, promote wound healing, and provide middle turbinate support. Absorbable biomaterials either provide clotting factors or a substrate to stimulate clotting. Other important characteristics of these agents include safety and efficacy, absorption kinetics, composition, usability (including form of the agent and delivery device), and cost. Biomaterials were extensively investigated and researched in the ear, nose, and throat literature well before the evolution of ESS, and this interest continues today. Both human and animal trials have contributed significantly to the understanding of these products and their role in ESS.

In an attempt to simplify the literature on biomaterials, this article is organized into effects on intraoperative hemostasis, postoperative hemostasis, and finally wound healing, in human studies and animal models. **Table 1** summarizes the literature on 20th century biomaterials and lists observations on hemostasis and wound healing in humans.

EFFECT OF 20TH CENTURY BIOMATERIALS ON HEMOSTASIS
Intraoperative Hemostasis

Absorbable porcine gelatin (Surgiflo, Ethicon Inc, Somerville, New Jersey) and thrombin combination; topical antifibrinolytics such as epsilon–aminocaproic acid (Amicar, Lederle Parenterals Inc, Carolina, Puerto Rico) and tranexamic acid (Cyklokapron, Pfizer, Puurs, Belgium); and hyaluronic acid have all been investigated in human studies for their intraoperative hemostatic properties after ESS. Surgiflo hemostatic matrix combined with thrombin is an absorbable porcine gelatin that was investigated by Woodworth and colleagues[14] after sinus surgery in a prospective trial. Results showed that patients experienced rapid hemostasis within 10 minutes, with a median time of 1 minute; however, this study had no control arm.[14]

Only one trial has studied topical antifibrinolytics after ESS. These agents prevent fibrinolysis and stabilize the blood clot. Results showed that topical epsilon–aminocaproic acid was ineffective at producing hemostasis compared with saline; however, tranexamic acid at low dose (100 mg) improved hemostasis significantly ($P<.05$). This observed effect was reduced at higher doses.[15] This study is only the second in the literature to use an objective surgical grade score to monitor hemostatic efficacy.

Table 1
Human studies on 20th century biomaterials

Biomaterial	Study	Study Design	Intraoperative Hemostasis	Postoperative Hemostasis	Adhesions/Wound Healing
Surgiflo/thrombin combination[14]	30 pts	Prospective (uncontrolled)	29/30 in 10 min	29/30 (1 req packing)	No adhesions
Epsilon–aminocaproic acid[15]	10 pts	DB RCT	Ineffective versus saline	10/10 pts	—
Tranexamic acid[15]	10 pts	DB RCT	Better versus saline (P<.05)	10/10 pts	—
Sepragel sinus[17]	20 pts	RCT	Same as no treatment	—	—
Quixil (fibrin glue)[8,16,69]	158 pts[8] 64 pts[16]	DB RCT[8] Prospective (controlled)[16]	Same as Merocel[8]		Same as Merocel[16]
Merocel[7,45]	16 pts[7] 61 pts[45]	Cohort[7] SB RCT[45]		16/16 pts[7]	No adhesions versus no packing (P = .001)[45]
Surgicel Nu-knit[18]	60 pts	RCT		60/60 pts, same as gauze and Merocel	—
MeroGel[22,43,44]	37 pts[22] 42 pts[44] 35 pts[43]	DB RCT[22] SB RCT[44] RCT[43]			Same as Merocel (3/37 adhesions)[22] Same as no pack[44] Same as removable pack[43]
Gelfilm[24,46]	115 pts[24] 51 pts[46]	Prospective (controlled)[24] RCT[46]			↑ adhesions verus MeroGel (P<.05)[24] ↑ granulations versus no pack (P<.05)[46]
Mitomycin C[23,49,50]	55 pts[49] 29 pts[23] 38 pts[50]	3 DB RCTs			All show same as no pack

Abbreviations: DB, double–blind; pts, patients; RCT, randomized controlled trial; req, required; SB, single–blind; ↑, increased; ↓, decreased.

Fibrin glue (Quixil, Omrix Co., Brussels, Belgium) is a combination of human thrombin and fibrinogen mixed with amino acids and salts, which allows this compound to form an easily applied gel. It was first used in the rhinology literature in the early 1990s, largely for managing cerebrospinal fluid rhinorrhea or for endonasal/transsphenoidal pituitary surgery. Vaiman and colleagues[16] showed that Quixil is effective in producing postoperative hemostasis, although they did not analyze how long it took to achieve.

Hyaluronic acid (Sepragel sinus, Genzyme Biosurgery, Cambridge, Massachusetts) is a viscoelastic gel containing polymers of highly purified forms of hyaluronic acid and has been investigated for immediate hemostasis by Frenkiel and colleagues.[17] Results showed no significant difference in total blood loss between the Sepragel sinus side and the no treatment side; however, a subjective general improvement of hemostasis was noted with the intervention side.

Postoperative Hemostasis

Surgiflo/thrombin combination, Merocel, and oxidized regenerated cellulose (Surgicel Nu-knit, Ethicon Inc, Somerville, New Jersey) have been studied for their effects on hemostasis after ESS. The Surgiflo/thrombin combination caused postoperative bleeding, requiring nasal packing in 1 of 30 patients.[14] Merocel was investigated in 16 patients after ESS, with no reported incidence of postoperative epistaxis.[7] Shinkwin and colleagues[18] compared Surgicel Nu-knit with Vaseline ribbon gauze and Merocel. All packing agents were equally effective with no incidence of postoperative epistaxis in any of the treatment arms.

Of particular interest is the number of patients experiencing postoperative epistaxis without any nasal packing or treatment at all. Athanasiadis and colleagues[15] found no incidence of postoperative epistaxis in 30 patients undergoing ESS. Jameson and colleagues[19] reported no incidence of postoperative epistaxis in 47 patients undergoing ESS without nasal packing. In a large retrospective review of patients after ESS, Orlandi and Lanza[20] challenged the practice of placing any pack at all, both in the immediate perioperative period and postoperatively. Among 165 patients, only 11.2% required nasal packing at the conclusion of operating, and none experienced postoperative epistaxis over 4 years.

Conclusions on Hemostatics

Tranexamic acid is an effective hemostatic option compared with no treatment, and fibrin glue is as effective as Merocel packing on immediate hemostasis. Sepragel sinus does not significantly reduce intraoperative blood loss when compared with no treatment. Additionally, one uncontrolled prospective trial suggests that Surgiflo/thrombin combination is effective in the immediate intraoperative period. In terms of postoperative bleeding, no evidence shows that any agent was more effective than no treatment at all; however, one large retrospective analysis suggests that immediate postoperative and long-term packing are not necessary in more than 90% of patients.

EFFECT OF 20TH CENTURY BIOMATERIALS ON ADHESION FORMATION

Adhesion formation is the most common complication encountered after ESS and can result in occlusion of the sinus drainage pathway. In addition, adhesions can result in recurrent symptoms and subsequent surgical failure. Studies have shown that up to 25% of patients who experience adhesion formation will require revision surgery in the future.[21] The incidence of adhesion formation after ESS is reported to be between 1% and 36%.[22–24] Therefore, a large body of literature is devoted to reducing the incidence of adhesion formation after ESS, with numerous biomaterials marketed for this effect.

When considering adhesion prevention, one must remember that agents that promote hemostasis through stimulation of the intrinsic coagulation cascade also stimulate inflammation.[25,26] Inflammatory responses are linked to hemostatic activation through a network of humoral and cellular components, including protease factors involved in the clotting and fibrinolytic cascades. Thus, the potential exists for potent coagulation cascade activation, leading to adverse wound healing.

Animal trials have also contributed significantly to the understanding of paranasal sinus wound healing and a large number of trials reflect this. The predominant models used are those involving sheep, rabbits, and mice. Sheep are an ideal model because they are large animals in which routine sinus surgical techniques can be used, and histologically their mucosa is identical to that of humans.[27]

Models of bacterial rhinosinusitis were developed using Merocel to block the maxillary sinus ostia, along with *Bacteroides fragilis* inoculation, resulting in a histologically confirmed, persistent, localized bacterial rhinosinusitis.[28] Finally, rabbits have well-pneumatized sinus cavities, and both their sinonasal anatomy and immunologic reactions are very similar to those of humans, making them a useful animal model for the study of biomaterials.[29]

Sheep Models

Shaw and colleagues[12] examined the effects of ribbon gauze packing and cottonoids on the nasal mucosa in a single-blind randomized controlled trial involving sheep. Nasal packing was left in situ for 10 minutes, followed by removal of packing and the associated mucosa. Blinded histologic analysis was then performed. Results showed that both packing agents produced more than a 50% loss of ciliated mucosal surface area ($P<.005$).

In a double-blind randomized controlled trial, McIntosh and colleagues compared the effects of Merocel (5 days) with no packing in the sheep model. Serial biopsies were taken at 4, 8, 12, and 16 weeks after treatment. Results showed no significant difference in the rate of reepithelialization, total surface ciliation, and overall maturity of cilia between the packed and non-packed sides at any point.[30]

Another further study compared the effects of MeroGel (Medtronic Xomed, Jacksonville, Florida) with no treatment in a sheep model of chronic sinusitis. This study created standardized mucosal injuries after histologic analysis of healing mucosa at 1, 2, 3, and 4 months postoperatively. Results showed no significant difference in adhesion formation or histologic features of reepithelialization, cilial height, and reciliation between the arms.[31]

The sheep model has also been used to examine the effects of drug delivery associated with nasal packing. Robinson and colleagues[32] studied the effects of prednisolone-impregnated MeroGel and MeroGel alone and found no difference. Finally, growth factors have also been shown to be important in epithelialization and collagen deposition, including insulin-like growth factor. Insulin-like growth factor–impregnated MeroGel was analyzed in the same sheep model after ESS and found to have a positive effect on mucosal regrowth and maturity in healthy sheep. However, when introduced in a model of chronic sinusitis, this effect was negated.[33]

Mice Models

Only one study used a murine model to examine the effects of biomaterials. Jacob and colleagues[34] conducted a randomized controlled trial involving 20 mice to evaluate the histologic effects of MeroGel. Results showed induced bone formation within the sino-nasal cavity, indicating that MeroGel may have osteogenic potential.

Rabbit Models

Maccabee and colleagues[35] studied the effects of MeroGel in six self-controlled rabbits through denuding the maxillary sinuses and performing histologic analysis of the regenerating mucosa. At 2 weeks postoperatively, the MeroGel sinuses showed extensive fibrosis compared with control sinuses, with minimal reabsorption of the biomaterial along with incorporation of the biomaterial within the regenerating mucosa. Proctor and colleagues[36] confirmed these findings, analyzing the effects of MeroGel in a rabbit model. Results showed that MeroGel caused significant stenosis of the ostia over a 2- to 3-week follow-up. Mitomycin C has also been investigated in the rabbit model, with one pilot study showing that increasing concentrations of Mito-mycin C can delay healing of an intranasal antrostomy (0.4 mg/mL, 1.0 mg/mL).[37]

Rahal and colleagues[38] confirmed these results. However, these trials were conducted in healthy rabbits without chronic rhinosinusitis, which may explain the discrepancies between these findings and those seen in human studies. Two published studies have investigated the effect of mucosa treated with retinoic acid (DPT Laboratories, San Antonio, Texas) in rabbits. Maccabee and colleagues[39] conducted a randomized controlled trial involving rabbits treated with retinoic acid, finding improved mucosal regeneration with less ciliary loss and fibrosis. These find-ings were also supported by Hwang and Chan,[40] again involving the healthy rabbit model.

Human Studies

Table 1 summarizes the data on adhesions and wound healing. MeroGel is a hyalur-onic acid, which is the major constituent of the extracellular matrix, and therefore acts as a scaffold for wound healing.[41] It has been shown to be the key factor in eliminating scarring in fetal wounds.[42] Franklin and Wright[43] also conducted a single-blind, randomized controlled trial to compare the effects of MeroGel and a nonabsorbable nasal packing (2–3 days), showing a trend toward improved postoperative endoscopic scores; however, this failed to reach significance at all time points. Additionally, Wormald and colleagues[44] investigated whether MeroGel had any effect on wound healing after ESS, showing no significant difference between the sides at 2, 4, and 8 weeks in the endoscopic features of adhesions, edema, or infection. Vaiman and colleagues[16] compared Quixil and Merocel, showing comparable results in the incidence of adhesion formation between the arms.

Miller and colleagues[22] compared Merocel pack (5–7 days) and hyaluronic acid (MeroGel). Patients underwent follow-up to 8 weeks postoperatively. Results showed both packing agents were associated with an 8% adhesion rate.[22] This finding contrasts with those of Vaiman and colleagues[16] and Pomerantz and Dutton,[7] which showed no evidence of adhesion formation with Merocel packing. Discrepancies between these studies maybe related to the timing of pack removal. Bugten and colleagues[45] investigated the effects of Merocel versus no nasal packing to determine whether removable nasal packing had any role after ESS. Video recordings taken 10 to 14 weeks after surgery showed 7 of 62 adhesions in the Merocel arm versus 29 of 54 adhesions in the no packing arm, a finding that was highly significant ($P = .001$).

Only one published article investigated the effects on wound healing of a combination of Surgiflo (Ferrosan, Soeborg, Denmark) and thrombin. This uncontrolled prospective trial involving 30 patients after ESS showed no incidence of reported adhesion formation. However, as indicated by the authors, further randomized controlled trials are indicated.[14]

Denatured porcine collagen (Gelfilm, Pharmacia and Upjohn Company, Kalamazoo, Michigan) has also been developed to reduce adhesion formation. It is an absorbable biomaterial manufactured from denatured porcine collagen. Results of two trials have shown adverse effects on wound healing, with one trial showing a significant increased in adhesions in patients implanted with Gelfilm compared with those implanted with MeroGel ($P<.05$),[24] and the second showing no significant difference in adhesion formation but a significant increase in granulation tissue formation in patients implanted with Gelfilm ($P<.05$).[46]

Mitomycin C is a topically applied agent that has been shown to reduce scar formation.[47] Additionally, it has been shown to inhibit nasal fibroblast proliferation and increase apoptosis.[48] It is isolated from the *Streptomyces caespitosus* strain of actinomyces, and used to crosslink DNA and inhibit cellular mitosis. Three human trials investigating the effects of mitomycin C against a saline control failed to show any significant findings regarding adhesion formation.[23,49,50]

Conclusions on Antiadhesion Effects of Biomaterials

No studies show that absorbable packing has any antiadhesion advantage over removable nasal packing or no packing at all. However, the same cannot be said for removable nasal packing, one single-blind randomized controlled trial showing a highly significant reduction in adhesion formation when Merocel is used. Three double-blind randomized controlled trials in the sheep model of chronic rhinosinusitis (CRS) confirm that MeroGel alone and with prednisolone or insulin-like growth factor has no effect on adhesion formation or cilial recovery. Two prospective, controlled rabbit trials suggested that MeroGel increases fibrosis and is incorporated within regenerating mucosa, and another showed that MeroGel displayed osteogenic potential.

Mitomycin C has shown promising results on healing ostia in two randomized controlled trials in the healthy rabbit model. However, these effects were not translated to patients who had post-ESS CRS, a conclusion also supported by Tabaee and colleagues.[51] Gelfilm stents have been shown to adversely affect the wound-healing process. One double-blind, randomized controlled trial shows that fibrin glue has no effect on adhesion formation, and one prospective trial suggests the same.

Finally, only one uncontrolled prospective trial has investigated the effects of the Surgiflo/thrombin combination, with no adhesions observed by the authors. Although the positive effects of vitamin A have been shown in healthy rabbit sinuses, further human trials are needed in patients who have CRS. Furthermore, although products containing oxidized regenerated cellulose (Surgicel) are widely known to have hemostatic properties,[6] and advocated as an absorbable nasal dressing after ESS,[18] no published literature has investigated their wound-healing properties after ESS.

20TH CENTURY BIOMATERIALS

An array of biomaterials are available. Several studies suggest that postoperative epistaxis is a rare event. In terms of immediate hemostasis, tranexamic acid and Surgiflo/thrombin combination have shown promising results. However, their wound-healing effects remain unknown. Although the effects of MeroGel on immediate hemostasis are unknown, human and animal trials show that it has no apparent positive effect on wound healing, and may worsen healing outcomes.

Sepragel sinus seems to have no objective effect on immediate hemostasis, and its effects on wound-healing are unknown. Mitomycin C has no effect on wound healing after ESS in patients. Finally, Gelfilm seems to potentially worsen healing outcomes and vitamin A shows promise in animal models only. The turn of the century clearly showed that a great need existed for the ideal biomaterial after ESS. Important characteristics of this product included the need to be effective in producing immediate and prolonged hemostasis, have no detrimental effect on wound healing, be absorbable and comfortable for patients, and, finally, have no risk for disease transmission.[7]

RECENT ADVANCES

Several recent advances and additions have been made to the biomaterial literature in recent years. Numerous additions to the already available biomaterials have been developed to meet the objectives of hemostatic properties and positive wound healing. FloSeal (Baxter International Inc, Deerfield, Illinois), carboxy-methyl-cellulose (AthroCare, Glenfield, United Kingdom), Platelet gel (PPAI Medical, Fort Myers, Florida), polyethylene glycol, microporous polysaccharide hemispheres (MPH, Medafor Inc, Minneapolis, Minnesota), and chitosan gel (Department of Chemistry, University of Otago, Dunedin, New Zealand) are all recent advances, developed with the hope of offering what no other product had previously offered.

FloSeal is a topical hemostatic agent consisting of gelatin matrix (bovine-derived) combined with human derived thrombin, and first became available to the market in 2000. Carboxymethylcellulose (CMC) nasal packing was developed in 2001, with its postulated ability to promote hemostasis by platelet aggregation.

Platelet gel is a fibrin tissue adhesive product manufactured from centrifugation of autologous whole blood, producing a platelet-rich plasma. It has the advantages of eliminating the risk for potential virus transmission and antibody formation to coagulation factors. Use in the rhinology community commenced in 2001, after a presentation to the American Rhinologic Society.

Microporous polysaccharide hemispheres (MPH) is a novel absorbable agent that is produced from purified potato starch, and acts to quickly extract fluids from blood, thereby concentrating serum proteins and platelets at the site of injury, and was approved for human use in 2006. A novel chitosan gel has also been recently developed from chitin, a natural biopolymer, and is postulated to achieve hemostasis through aggregation of erythrocytes. It also has been shown to have an inhibitory effect on fibroblast proliferation.[52,53]

No published literature has investigated the hemostatic or wound-healing properties of polyethylene glycol (NasoPore, Polyganics B.V., Groningen, The Netherlands) after ESS. All other products have recently been investigated in both human and animal trials, importantly in the area of hemostasis and wound healing. **Table 2** summarizes the data regarding human trials on these 21st century biomaterials.

EFFECT OF 21ST CENTURY BIOMATERIALS ON HEMOSTASIS
Intraoperative Hemostasis

Gall and colleagues[54] found that FloSeal was effective in producing hemostasis in 17 of 18 patients, and also found that the average time to hemostasis was 2 minutes. Additionally, Jameson and colleagues[19] showed that the FloSeal group had a significantly faster time to hemostasis (16.4 minutes) than the control group (30.8 minutes). Baumann and colleagues[55] compared FloSeal with Merocel in a nonrandomized trial, and found that intraoperative hemostasis occurred within 3 minutes in both arms. Significant variability is shown between these studies on the time to hemostasis.

Table 2
Human studies on 21st century biomaterials

Biomaterial	Study	Study Design	Intraoperative Hemostasis	Postoperative Hemostasis	Adhesions/Wound Healing
FloSeal[13,19,21,54,55]	18 pts[54]	Prospective (uncontrolled)[54]	Rapid hemostasis 17/18 pts[54] (P = .028[19])	17/18 pts (1 req packing)[54] same as Merocel[55]	↑ adhesions and granulations (P = .006)[13] ↑ adhesions (P = .009)[21] No effect (same as removable pack)[19]
	45 pts[19]	DB RCT[19]			
	50 pts[55]	DB RCT[55]			
	20 pts[13]	DB RCT[13]			
	172 pts[21]	Retrospective[21]			
MPH[56,60]	65 pts[56]	Prospective (uncontrolled)[56]	Rapid hemostasis (30–45 s)[56]	65/65 pts,[56] less bleeding on POD#1 versus untreated side[60]	8/65 adhesions[56]
	40 pts[60]	SB RCT[60]			
Platelet gel[7]	16 pts	Prospective		16/16 pts (same as Merocel)	No adhesions (same as Merocel)
CMC mesh[58,59,62]	15 pts[58]	Prospective (uncontrolled)[58]	20% persistent bleeding[58]	15/15 pts[58] 41/41 pts (same as no pack)[59]	No adhesions[58] No effect (same as no pack)[62]
CMC gel[59,62]	41 pts[59]	SB RCT[59]			

Abbreviations: DB, double–blind; pts, patients; RCT, randomized controlled trial; req, required; SB, single–blind; ↑, increased; ↓, decreased.

One recent study investigating the effects of MPH on hemostasis showed that hemostasis occurred between 30 and 45 seconds after application.[56] Finally, Valentine and colleagues[57] conducted a randomized controlled trial into the efficacy of chitosan gel in producing hemostasis in the sheep model of CRS. This study involved a standardized wound injury, followed by application of chitosan gel to one nasal cavity, with the opposite acting as a control. The Boezaart bleeding scale was taken at 2-minute intervals to objectively evaluate hemostatic efficacy. Results showed that the chitosan gel side was significantly more hemostatic at 2, 4, and 6 minutes after injury (P<.05). Complete hemostasis occurred by 6 minutes for all chitosan gel sides; however, control side bleeding was noted on three sides at 8 minutes and one at 10 minutes.[57]

Postoperative Hemostasis

When comparing FloSeal and Merocel after ESS, the incidence of postoperative epistaxis was similar (ie, 1 among 50 versus 2 among 50), indicating that these were equally as effective.[55] However, removable nasal packing causes bleeding on removal, and when this was taken into consideration, a significantly greater number of bleeds was noted in the Merocel group (21.87%; P<.001).[16] Gall and colleagues[54] noted that 1 of 18 patients required nasal packing 6 hours after FloSeal application for persistent epistaxis postoperatively. Pomerantz and Dutton[7] reported no incidence of postoperative epistaxis in either the Platelet gel or Merocel arm.

Two studies reported on CMC's efficacy on hemostasis postoperatively. In an uncontrolled pilot study by Karkos and colleagues,[58] nursing staff reported persistent oozing in 20% of patients treated with CMC mesh; however, no patient required intervention. Kastl and colleagues[59] showed that CMC mesh had no significant effect on postoperative bleeding. No episodes of postoperative epistaxis were reported in 65 patients treated with MPH after ESS.[56]

In a randomized controlled trial evaluating MPH, 40 patients who had CRS underwent ESS and had only one side treated with MPH (with the opposite side serving as a control) at the conclusion of surgery. Patients were blinded to side of treatment, and the results showed that MPH significantly reduced bleeding (compared with the untreated side; P = .001) during the early recovery period after ESS.[60]

Conclusions on Hemostatics

FloSeal produces rapid hemostasis compared with control. Both studies investigating CMC seem to suggest that CMC mesh has no significant effect on postoperative bleeding. The effects of MPH after ESS have been reported in an observational study and in one prospective, randomized, controlled trial, and have shown efficacy in reducing postoperative bleeding. One randomized controlled trial investigates the efficacy of Chitosan gel, and shows rapid hemostasis in the sheep model of ESS.

EFFECT OF 21ST CENTURY BIOMATERIALS ON ADHESION FORMATION
Human Studies

Chandra and colleagues[61] investigated the wound-healing effects of FloSeal by comparing FloSeal versus thrombin-soaked Gelfoam (Pharmacia and Upjohn Company, Kalamazoo, Michigan). Patients were followed up at 1 and 6 weeks postoperatively. Results showed that the mean adhesion score was increased in the FloSeal side, a highly significant finding (P = .006). Adhesions developed on 11 sides treated with FloSeal, compared with only 2 of the sides treated with Gelfoam.

Similar findings were noted for granulation tissue formation ($P = .007$). Follow-up of these patients occurred for an average of 21 months after surgery and showed that 56% of FloSeal sides had an adhesion, compared with 11% of the thrombin-soaked Gelfoam sides ($P = .013$). Of the sides treated with Gelfoam, 28% required lysis versus none of the thrombin-soaked Gelfoam sides ($P = .046$). Histologic examination of an adhesion on the FloSeal side showed incorporation of the foreign material.[61]

Shrime and colleagues[21] attempted to determine the incidence, outcomes, and risk factors for adhesion formation after ESS with middle turbinate medialization with and without FloSeal. A statistically significant higher incidence of adhesion formation was noted in patients who underwent treatment with FloSeal (18.9%) versus those who received no packing (6.7%; $P = .009$).[21]

Statistical multivariate analysis comparing adhesion formation and surgical and demographic variables showed a statistically significant correlation only with the FloSeal ($P = .0063$; odds ratio, 5.3330; 95% CI, 1.61–17.71).[21] Explanation for this effect maybe the bidirectional relationship between coagulation and inflammation, wherein strong initiation of the coagulation cascade results in strong activation of inflammation and fibrosis.[26]

These results contrast with the findings of Jameson and colleagues,[19] who showed no significant difference between sides in 45 patients enrolled, which are similar results to those of a retrospective analysis by Pomerantz and Dutton,[7] who compared platelet gel and Merocel and found no incidence of adhesion formation in either arm, or evidence of exuberant granulation tissue.

Postoperative adhesion formation was not observed in a pilot study with the use of CMC mesh.[58] Kastl and colleagues[62] conducted a randomized controlled trial comparing the effects of CMC mesh, CMC gel, and no nasal packing in 26 patients after ESS. All patients acted as their own control. Results showed no significant clinical effect on wound healing. Sindwani[56] continued his observation of 65 patients who underwent treatment with MPH after ESS, and found a 12.3% incidence of adhesion formation; however, no control group was used for comparison.

Sheep Models

One study has investigated the efficacy of chitosan gel on mucosal wound healing after ESS in the sheep model of CRS. Athanasiadis and colleagues[63] conducted a double-blind randomized controlled trial involving 20 sheep infested with nasal bot fly (causing an eosinophilic sinusitis). Standardized mucosal injuries were created, followed by the application of either chitosan gel, polyethylene glycol (SprayGel, Confluent Surgical, Waltham, Massachusetts), recombinant tissue factor (rTF, Dade Innovin, Marburg, Germany), or no treatment. Histologic analysis of mucosal biopsies was then performed, with results showing that chitosan gel significantly decreased adhesion formation compared with rTF, with a noticeable trend when compared with SprayGel and control (14% versus 0% and 40% versus 0%, respectively). Chitosan gel significantly improved reepithelialization, reciliation, and cilial grade ($P<.05$).[63]

Rabbit Models

Maccabee and colleagues[35] studied the effects of FloSeal in six self-controlled rabbits by denuding the maxillary sinuses and performing histologic analysis of the regenerating mucosa. At 2 weeks postoperatively, FloSeal sinuses showed extensive fibrosis when compared with control sinuses, with minimal reabsorption of the biomaterial along with incorporation of the biomaterial within the regenerating mucosa.

Antisdel and colleagues[64] conducted a single-blind randomized controlled trial investigating the effects of microporous polysaccharide hemispheres versus FloSeal in 14 self-controlled rabbits. Ten rabbits underwent bilateral maxillary sinus stripping, with five receiving unilateral FloSeal placement and five receiving unilateral MPH placement (opposite side acting as control). An additional two animals underwent unilateral FloSeal placement in an unstripped maxillary sinus, and two animals underwent unilateral MPH placement (opposite side acting as control).

Results showed no significant changes in MPH-treated sinuses compared with respective controls; however, FloSeal sides showed extensive loss of cilia, inflammation, and fibrosis, both in the denuded and mucosa intact sinuses,[64] a finding consistent with that of Maccabee and colleagues.[35]

Conclusions on Antiadhesion Effects of Biomaterials

To conclude on the effects of FloSeal on regenerating mucosa, one double-blind randomized controlled trial shows increased adhesion formation and granulations,[13] with this finding confirmed by a large retrospective case series.[21] Again, the rabbit model has shown that FloSeal increases fibrosis and is incorporated within the healing mucosa, a finding supported by a second independent study.[35,64]

CMC mesh and gel seem to have no appreciable effect on postoperative wound healing compared with no treatment.[62] MPH seems to have an adhesion incidence comparable to that reported by most endoscopic sinus surgeons.[56] Additionally, MPH has no appreciable detrimental effect on mucosal healing in the rabbit model.[64] Finally, chitosan gel, in the sheep model of chronic rhinosinusitis, significantly improves microscopic features of wound healing and reduces adhesion formation after ESS.[63]

CONCERNS AND CONCLUSIONS

Recent advances in the biomaterial literature has seen the addition of several agents, including those containing bovine or human blood products to exploit the intrinsic and extrinsic coagulation cascades for producing hemostasis. FloSeal, although an effective hemostatic agent, seems to have detrimental effects on wound healing in patients post-ESS and in animal models. Fibrin glue also seems to be effective against immediate bleeding after ESS.

Platelet gel seems to be equally effective as Merocel in its abilities to maintain hemostasis, and the only published trial after ESS shows no incidence of adhesion formation with either product. However, ongoing concern exists regarding antibody formation and disease transmission of thrombin, fibrin, and collagen products, limiting their usefulness in ESS.[16,65–67]

Dorion and colleagues[66] reviewed the use of topical bovine thrombin preparation in 120 surgical patients. They found that between 5% and 15% of exposed patients developed antibodies to coagulations factors, and those exposed more than once were eight times more likely to develop antibodies. They also noted a 1.7% risk for developing serious bleeding complications from exposure to bovine thrombin.[66] In addition, the theoretical risk exists for infectious disease transmission of HIV, hepatitis, and Creutzfeldt-Jakob disease, all possible with blood products.[68]

MPH and chitosan gel have recently entered the literature, both having the advantage of conferring no risk for disease transmission. Findings suggest that MPH has an attractive role in producing immediate intraoperative hemostasis, with one prospective randomized study showing efficacy in reducing postoperative bleeding during the early recovery period after surgery. A study using the rabbit model suggests that this substance does not interfere with normal mucosal regeneration and wound healing.

Only one product in the rhinology literature has shown positive effects in both wound healing and immediate hemostasis. Chitosan gel has been shown in the CRS sheep model of ESS to have produced rapid hemostasis after application and has been shown to significantly improve the microscopic features of wound healing and reduce adhesion formation after ESS in an animal model. Newer 21st century agents offer distinct advantages because of their unique composition and rapid clearance profiles. The selection of packing material for any given sinus procedure should be based on surgeon preference and the details of the specific case.

REFERENCES

1. von Schoenberg M, Robinson P, Ryan R. Nasal packing after routine nasal surgery—is it justified? J Laryngol Otol 1993;107:902–5.
2. Samad I, Stevens HE, Maloney A. The efficacy of nasal septal surgery. J Otolaryngol 1992;21:88–91.
3. Kennedy DW. Functional endoscopic sinus surgery. Technique. Arch Otolaryngol 1985;111:643–9.
4. Kennedy DW. Middle turbinate resection: evaluating the issues–should we resect normal middle turbinates? Arch Otolaryngol Head Neck Surg 1998;124:107.
5. Stevens RW. Nasal packing; the rubber pneumatic pack. AMA Arch Otolaryngol 1951;54:191–4.
6. Huggins S. Control of hemorrhage in otorhinolaryngologic surgery with oxidized regenerated cellulose. Eye Ear Nose Throat Mon 1969;48:420–3.
7. Pomerantz J, Dutton JM. Platelet gel for endoscopic sinus surgery. Ann Otol Rhinol Laryngol 2005;114:699–704.
8. Vaiman M, Eviatar E, Segal S. Effectiveness of second-generation fibrin glue in endonasal operations. Otolaryngol Head Neck Surg 2002;126:388–91.
9. Vaiman M, Eviatar E, Segal S. The use of fibrin glue as hemostatic in endonasal operations: a prospective, randomized study. Rhinology 2002;40:185–8.
10. Weber R, Keerl R, Hochapfel F, et al. Packing in endonasal surgery. Am J Otolaryngol 2001;22:306–20.
11. Weber R, Hochapfel F, Draf W. Packing and stents in endonasal surgery. Rhinology 2000;38:49–62.
12. Shaw CL, Dymock RB, Cowin A, et al. Effect of packing on nasal mucosa of sheep. J Laryngol Otol 2000;114:506–9.
13. Chandra RK, Conley DB, Kern RC. The effect of FloSeal on mucosal healing after endoscopic sinus surgery: a comparison with thrombin-soaked gelatin foam. Am J Rhinol 2003;17:51–5.
14. Woodworth BA, Chandra RK, LeBenger JD, et al. A gelatin-thrombin matrix for hemostasis after endoscopic sinus surgery. Am J Otolaryngol 2009;30:49–53.
15. Athanasiadis T, Beule AG, Wormald PJ. Effects of topical antifibrinolytics in endoscopic sinus surgery: a pilot randomized controlled trial. Am J Rhinol 2007;21:737–42.
16. Vaiman M, Eviatar E, Shlamkovich N, et al. Use of fibrin glue as a hemostatic in endoscopic sinus surgery. Ann Otol Rhinol Laryngol 2005;114:237–41.
17. Frenkiel S, Desrosiers MY, Nachtigal D. Use of hylan B gel as a wound dressing after endoscopic sinus surgery. J Otolaryngol 2002;31(Suppl 1):S41–4.
18. Shinkwin CA, Beasley N, Simo R, et al. Evaluation of Surgicel Nu-knit, Merocel and Vasolene gauze nasal packs: a randomized trial. Rhinology 1996;34:41–3.

19. Jameson M, Gross CW, Kountakis SE. FloSeal use in endoscopic sinus surgery: effect on postoperative bleeding and synechiae formation. Am J Otolaryngol 2006;27(2):86–90.
20. Orlandi RR, Lanza DC. Is nasal packing necessary following endoscopic sinus surgery? Laryngoscope 2004;114:1541–4.
21. Shrime MG, Tabaee A, Hsu AK, et al. Synechia formation after endoscopic sinus surgery and middle turbinate medialization with and without FloSeal. Am J Rhinol 2007;21(2):174–9.
22. Miller RS, Steward DL, Tami TA, et al. The clinical effects of hyaluronic acid ester nasal dressing (Merogel) on intranasal wound healing after functional endoscopic sinus surgery. Otolaryngol Head Neck Surg 2003;128:862–9.
23. Anand VK, Tabaee A, Kacker A, et al. The role of mitomycin C in preventing synechia and stenosis after endoscopic sinus surgery. Am J Rhinol 2004;18:311–4.
24. Catalano PJ, Roffman EJ. Evaluation of middle meatal stenting after minimally invasive sinus techniques (MIST). Otolaryngol Head Neck Surg 2003;128: 875–81.
25. Levi M, van der Poll T. Two-way interactions between inflammation and coagulation. Trends Cardiovasc Med 2005;15:254–9.
26. Levi M, van der Poll T, Buller HR. Bidirectional relation between inflammation and coagulation. Circulation 2004;109:2698–704.
27. Illum L. Nasal delivery. The use of animal models to predict performance in man. J Drug Target 1996;3:427–42.
28. Jacob A, Faddis BT, Chole RA. Chronic bacterial rhinosinusitis: description of a mouse model. Arch Otolaryngol Head Neck Surg 2001;127:657–64.
29. Liang KL, Jiang RS, Wang J, et al. Developing a rabbit model of rhinogenic chronic rhinosinusitis. Laryngoscope 2008;118:1076–81.
30. McIntosh D, Cowin A, Adams D, et al. The effect of an expandable polyvinyl acetate (Merocel) pack on the healing of the nasal mucosa of sheep. Am J Rhinol 2005;19:577–81.
31. Rajapaksa SP, Cowin A, Adams D, et al. The effect of a hyaluronic acid-based nasal pack on mucosal healing in a sheep model of sinusitis. Am J Rhinol 2005;19:572–6.
32. Robinson S, Adams D, Wormald PJ. The effect of nasal packing and prednisolone on mucosal healing and reciliation in a sheep model. Rhinology 2004; 42(2):68–72.
33. Rajapaksa S, McIntosh D, Cowin A, et al. The effect of insulin-like growth factor 1 incorporated into a hyaluronic acid-based nasal pack on nasal mucosal healing in a healthy sheep model and a sheep model of chronic sinusitis. Am J Rhinol 2005;19:251–6.
34. Jacob A, Faddis BT, Chole RA. MeroGel hyaluronic acid sinonasal implants: osteogenic implications. Laryngoscope 2002;112:37–42.
35. Maccabee MS, Trune DR, Hwang PH. Effects of topically applied biomaterials on paranasal sinus mucosal healing. Am J Rhinol 2003;17:203–7.
36. Proctor M, Proctor K, Shu XZ, et al. Composition of hyaluronan affects wound healing in the rabbit maxillary sinus. Am J Rhinol 2006;20:206–11.
37. Ingrams DR, Volk MS, Biesman BS, et al. Sinus surgery: does mitomycin C reduce stenosis? Laryngoscope 1998;108:883–6.
38. Rahal A, Peloquin L, Ahmarani C. Mitomycin C in sinus surgery: preliminary results in a rabbit model. J Otolaryngol 2001;30:1–5.
39. Maccabee MS, Trune DR, Hwang PH. Paranasal sinus mucosal regeneration: the effect of topical retinoic acid. Am J Rhinol 2003;17:133–7.

40. Hwang PH, Chan JM. Retinoic acid improves ciliogenesis after surgery of the maxillary sinus in rabbits. Laryngoscope 2006;116:1080–5.

41. Chen WY, Abatangelo G. Functions of hyaluronan in wound repair. Wound Repair Regen 1999;7:79–89.

42. Samuels P, Tan AK. Fetal scarless wound healing. J Otolaryngol 1999;28: 296–302.

43. Franklin JH, Wright ED. Randomized, controlled, study of absorbable nasal packing on outcomes of surgical treatment of rhinosinusitis with polyposis. Am J Rhinol 2007;21:214–7.

44. Wormald PJ, Boustred RN, Le T, et al. A prospective single-blind randomized controlled study of use of hyaluronic acid nasal packs in patients after endoscopic sinus surgery. Am J Rhinol 2006;20:7–10.

45. Bugten V, Nordgard S, Skogvoll E, et al. Effects of nonabsorbable packing in middle meatus after sinus surgery. Laryngoscope 2006;116:83–8.

46. Tom LW, Palasti S, Potsic WP, et al. The effects of gelatin film stents in the middle meatus. Am J Rhinol 1997;11:229–32.

47. Kao SC, Liao CL, Tseng JH, et al. Dacryocystorhinostomy with intraoperative mitomycin C. Ophthalmology 1997;104:86–91.

48. Hu D, Sires BS, Tong DC, et al. Effect of brief exposure to mitomycin C on cultured human nasal mucosa fibroblasts. Ophthal Plast Reconstr Surg 2000; 16:119–25.

49. Chung JH, Cosenza MJ, Rahbar R, et al. Mitomycin C for the prevention of adhesion formation after endoscopic sinus surgery: a randomized, controlled study. Otolaryngol Head Neck Surg 2002;126:468–74.

50. Chan KO, Gervais M, Tsaparas Y, et al. Effectiveness of intraoperative mitomycin C in maintaining the patency of a frontal sinusotomy: a preliminary report of a double-blind randomized placebo-controlled trial. Am J Rhinol 2006;20:295–9.

51. Tabaee A, Brown SM, Anand VK. Mitomycin C and endoscopic sinus surgery: where are we? Curr Opin Otolaryngol Head Neck Surg 2007;15:40–3.

52. Zhou J, Liwski RS, Elson C, et al. Reduction in postsurgical adhesion formation after cardiac surgery in a rabbit model using N, O-carboxymethyl chitosan to block cell adherence. J Thorac Cardiovasc Surg 2008;135:777–83.

53. Xia CS, Hong GX, Dou RR, et al. Effects of chitosan on cell proliferation and collagen production of tendon sheath fibroblasts, epitenon tenocytes, and endotenon tenocytes. Chin J Traumatol 2005;8:369–74.

54. Gall RM, Witterick IJ, Shargill NS, et al. Control of bleeding in endoscopic sinus surgery: use of a novel gelatin-based hemostatic agent. J Otolaryngol 2002;31: 271–4.

55. Baumann A, Caversaccio M. Hemostasis in endoscopic sinus surgery using a specific gelatin-thrombin based agent (FloSeal). Rhinology 2003;41:244–9.

56. Sindwani R. Use of novel hemostatic powder MPH for endoscopic sinus surgery: Initial impressions. Otolaryngol Head Neck Surg 2009;140:262–3.

57. Valentine R, Athanasiadis T, Moratti S, et al. The efficacy of a novel chitosan gel on hemostasis after endoscopic sinus surgery in a sheep model of chronic rhinosinusitis. Am J Rhinol Allergy 2009;23(1):71–5.

58. Karkos PD, Thinakararajan T, Goodyear P, et al. Day-case endoscopic sinus surgery using dissolvable haemostatic nasal packs: a pilot study. Eur Arch Otorhinolaryngol 2007;264:1171–4.

59. Kastl KG, Betz CS, Siedek V, et al. Control of bleeding following functional endoscopic sinus surgery using carboxy-methylated cellulose packing. Eur Arch Otorhinolaryngol 2009;266(8):1239–43.

60. Antisdel JL, West-Denning R, Sindwani R. Effect of microporous polysaccharide hemospheres (mph) on bleeding after endoscopic sinus surgery: prospective randomized controlled study. Otolaryngol Head Neck Surg 2009;141:353–7.
61. Chandra RK, Conley DB, Haines GK 3rd, et al. Long-term effects of FloSeal packing after endoscopic sinus surgery. Am J Rhinol 2005;19:240–3.
62. Kastl KG, Betz CS, Siedek V, et al. Effect of carboxymethylcellulose nasal packing on wound healing after functional endoscopic sinus surgery. Am J Rhinol Allergy 2009;23:80–4.
63. Athanasiadis T, Beule AG, Robinson BH, et al. Effects of a novel chitosan gel on mucosal wound healing following endoscopic sinus surgery in a sheep model of chronic rhinosinusitis. Laryngoscope 2008;118:1088–94.
64. Antisdel JL, Janney CG, Long JP, et al. Hemostatic agent microporous polysaccharide hemospheres (MPH) does not affect healing or intact sinus mucosa. Laryngoscope 2008;118:1265–9.
65. Green D. Spontaneous inhibitors to coagulation factors. Clin Lab Haematol 2000; 22(Suppl 1):21–5.
66. Dorion RP, Hamati HF, Landis B, et al. Risk and clinical significance of developing antibodies induced by topical thrombin preparations. Arch Pathol Lab Med 1998; 122:887–94.
67. Flaherty MJ, Henderson R, Wener MH. Iatrogenic immunization with bovine thrombin: a mechanism for prolonged thrombin times after surgery. Ann Intern Med 1989;111:631–4.
68. Dresdale A, Rose EA, Jeevanandam V, et al. Preparation of fibrin glue from single-donor fresh-frozen plasma. Surgery 1985;97:750–5.
69. Vaiman M, Sarfaty S, Shlamkovich N, et al. Fibrin sealant: alternative to nasal packing in endonasal operations. A prospective randomized study. Isr Med Assoc J 2005;7:571–4.

Local Drug Delivery

Richard J. Harvey, MD[a],*, Rodney J. Schlosser, MD[b]

KEYWORDS

- Sinus surgery • Topical • Irrigation • Spray • Steroid
- Surfactant • Mucoadhesion

Respiratory epithelial damage, mucus hypersecretion, mucociliary dysfunction, and the release of proinflammatory products at the sinus mucosa all mediate the prolonged inflammation of chronic rhinosinusitis (CRS).[1] The perceived role of local microbial flora in CRS has evolved from one of causation to disease modifer.[2] Although there has been a shift to anti-inflammatory therapies in CRS,[3,4] bacteria and fungi are still likely to be powerful mediators of inflammation. The current model of CRS pathophysiology focuses on the interaction of the inflammatory mucosal disease with microbial flora and the failure of the mechanical and innate immunity (**Fig. 1**). Current systemic agents, such as oral or intravenous antimicrobials or anti-inflammatories, have significant side effects and are not successful in many patients. This problem has led rhinologists to examine local delivery of topical therapies. These treatment strategies are important in the management of the disordered inflammation of CRS, and are likely to be pivotal to modifying the expanding pathologic mechanisms that mediate this disease.

The general therapeutic goal of topical management may also lie between potentially competing actions of mechanical lavage and pharmaceutical intervention. The mechanical removal of mucus, antigen, pollutants, inflammatory products, and bacteria/biofilms is often targeted with topical approaches. These interventions rely on high-volume positive pressure solutions to provide shearing forces with additives to alter air-surface-liquid (ASL) tension. However, the same approach may not be appropriate for delivery of pharmaceutical preparations. Complete sinus distribution, prolonged mucosal contact time with local absorption, and minimal wastage are often the desired properties. There is currently a wide array of antimicrobial, anti-inflammatory and immunomodulatory agents being investigated for CRS, which are beyond the scope of this article. The discussion here focuses on modern concepts in local drug therapy, for the macroscopic factors that affect distribution within the sinonasal system and those factors within the microenvironment that influence absorption (**Table 1**).

[a] Rhinology and Skull Base Surgery, Department of Otolaryngology/Skull Base Surgery, St Vincent's Hospital, 354 Victoria Street, Darlinghurst, Sydney, NSW 2010, Australia
[b] Rhinology and Skull Base Surgery, Department of Otolaryngology/Head & Neck Surgery, Medical University of South Carolina, 135 Rutledge Avenue, Charleston, SC 29425, USA
* Corresponding author.
E-mail address: richard@sydneyentclinic.com (R.J. Harvey).

Otolaryngol Clin N Am 42 (2009) 829–845
doi:10.1016/j.otc.2009.07.005

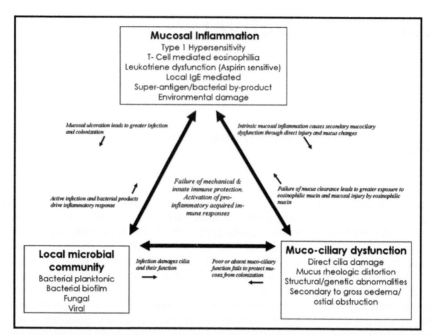

Fig. 1. Pathophysiologic interaction of intrinsic mucosal inflammation, microbial flora, and mucociliary dysfunction. Current topical therapies can affect all 3 interacting processes: the ability to substitute for loss of mucociliary clearance and alter mucus rheology, delivery of steroids to intrinsic mucosal inflammation, and antimicrobial therapies. (*Courtesy of* Division of Rhinology, St Vincent's Hospital; with permission.)

MACRODELIVERY

The ability of the drug to reach the appropriate anatomic region in the paranasal system will always be important, and has been the subject of much research in the past 5 years. Delivery techniques, surgical state of the sinus cavity, delivery device, and fluid dynamics (volume, pressure, position) have a significant impact on the delivery of topical therapies to the sinus mucosa.

Sinus Surgery

Distribution of topical solution to the unoperated sinuses is limited,[5] and in the setting of CRS with mucosal edema it is probably only on the order of less than 2% of total

Table 1	
Factors influencing mucosal drug delivery	
Local Absorption (Micro)	**Sinonasal Distribution (Macro)**
Mucus blanket	Surgical state
Mechanical obstruction to diffusion	Device
Cell surface charge	Position
Mucin and protein binding	Volume
Mucociliary clearance	Pressure
Mucosal residence time	Anatomic dimensions of surgical cavity

irrigation volume.[6] Nebulization is also ineffective, with less than 3% sinus penetration.[7] A fundamentally held belief among those treating CRS patients is that endoscopic sinus surgery (ESS) improves the delivery of topical medications to the sinonasal mucosa,[8,9] yet only recent evidence exists to support this claim.[5,10] Endoscopic sinus surgery is essential to effectively allow topical distribution to the sinuses. The frontal and sphenoid sinus are essentially inaccessible before surgery (**Fig. 2**)[5] and an ostial size of greater than 4 mm is required to even begin seeing penetration to the maxillary sinus.[10] For those with mucosal edema and chronic inflammation, distribution is probably worse.[6] In medically managing CRS, the use of expensive and time-wasting topical therapies, such as increasing topical steroid options (**Fig. 3**), are probably not supported prior to ESS.

There is growing evidence that a predominant feature of CRS is a shift in mucosal immune response to a proinflammatory process, whether Th1 or Th2 dominated. This process differs from the normal mechanical and innate immunity that provides stable, healthy mucosa.[2] Due to their anti-inflammatory action, corticosteroids have long been the drug of choice for this purpose, and are one of the most widely studied pharmacologic agents. Unfortunately, the evidence for a role of nasal steroids in the management of CRS is weak. Most studies include unoperated patients or a mix of pre- and postsurgical populations. This patient selection raises greater questions of what mucosa one is actually treating in these studies.

The potential for observing a focal effect on secondary turbinate reactivity in CRS without any actual impact on the sinus mucosa is great. Steroid sprays in unoperated patients leads to almost no sinus distribution,[5,11] so it is not surprising that researchers using steroid postoperatively with direct application to the sinus mucosa have demonstrated benefit,[12–14] and those with a mixed or unoperated population have found less benefit.[15,16] In addition, there is a significant difference in the way in which ESS is delivered across institutions, as some post-ESS cavities are opened widely, whereas other surgeons practice techniques to simply dilate or create very conservative sinusotomies (**Fig. 4**). The heterogeneous group of surgical comparisons makes evaluating locally delivered therapies even more difficult to assess,[17] and minimal techniques have proliferated without consideration of many of these factors.[18]

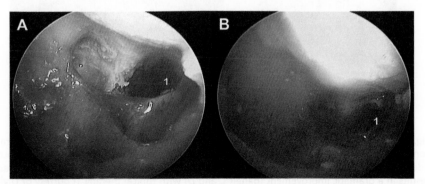

Fig. 2. (*A, B*) Images taken from intrafrontal sinus video. Even after endoscopic sinus surgery (ESS) (*A*), the frontal recess (1) is not well penetrated with simple delivery. Only with head-down positioning, high volume, and positive pressure irrigation does frontal sinus delivery occur.

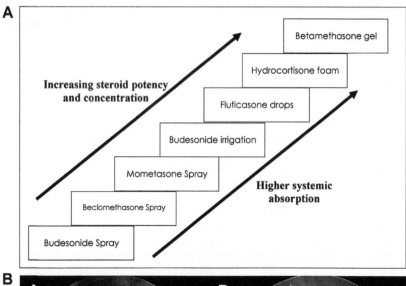

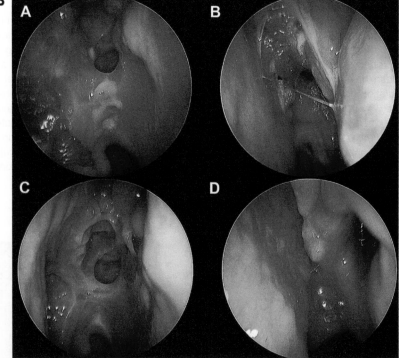

Fig. 3. (A) The authors' current local steroid potency ladder. Patients rarely go past mometasone spray before surgery. The drug simply does not reach the sinus mucosa without adequate exposure from surgery. (B) Postsurgical disease (panels A and B), however, often results in a dramatic improvement (panels C and D) with topical therapy. (Courtesy of Division of Rhinology, St Vincent's Hospital; with permission.)

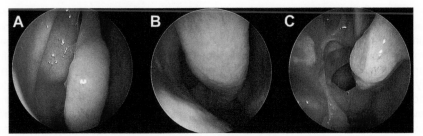

Fig. 4. Appearance of the right middle meatus after surgery. (*A*) Ostial dilatation. (*B*) Mini ESS. (*C*) Formal ESS. The potential difference in assisting topical delivery to the sinus mucosa is great, thus making studies using a heterogeneous group of such patients very difficult to interpret.

Delivery Devices

Nebulizers poorly penetrate the sinuses even after maximal ESS,[19] and large-volume squeeze bottles or passive flow devices seem to have the best efficacy post ESS.[5,8,9,19] Presurgery, the distribution to the sinuses is extremely limited regardless of device,[5,6,10] and sprays are the least effective of all (**Fig. 5**).[5] Neti pots have advantage in the unoperated sinus, as head position and retrograde flow allows some

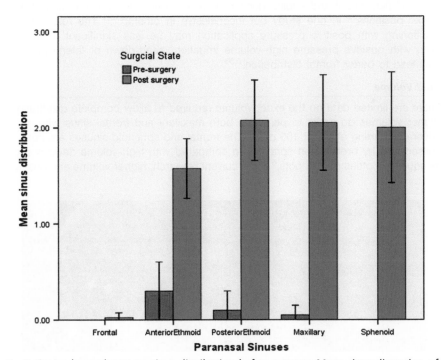

Fig. 5. Sprays have almost no sinus distribution before surgery. Mean sinus dispersion of radiographic contrast is extremely limited without surgical exposure of the sinus mucosa. In the frontal and sphenoid sinuses, this is especially true. (*Courtesy of* Division of Rhinology, St Vincent's Hospital; with permission.)

penetration.[5] Postsurgery distribution is superior with high-volume positive pressure devices.[5,10,20] Research into topical distribution often quantifies penetration and surface area covered but not volume, shearing forces, or mucosal contact time. From intrasinus video observation during the authors' studies, there is a very significant difference in fluid dynamics between irrigation techniques that is difficult to quantify. Simple computed tomography studies or endoscopic grading do not take into account the increased hydrostatic forces seen with large-volume positive pressure devices, such as a squeeze bottle, when compared with large-volume, low-pressure devices such as the Neti pot (**Fig. 6**). In addition, it is unknown whether these increased irrigation pressures are beneficial. Simple low-volume sprays and drops have very poor distribution and should be considered a nasal cavity treatment only, especially before ESS.[5] Although multiple devices and head positions have been trialed, less than 50% of most low-volume applications will reach even the middle meatus.[21]

Position for Sinus Fluid Delivery

There are incomplete data on the most effective positioning for delivering fluid to the nasal cavity and paranasal sinuses.[5,21–29] The majority of these studies involve assessment of dye "around" the middle turbinate with simple sprays and drops in presurgical patients. Many commercial products recommend a head-down, over sink, with nose to ground position for irrigation. This orientation is practical and makes runoff easy to collect. Evidence for the efficacy in delivery of drops to the middle meatus relative to head position demonstrates that the "Mygind" and "Ragan" (left lateral and supine positions) were superior to "Mecca" and "Head Back" positions[22] in one study but inconclusive in others.[21,29] The relevance of positioning with positive pressure application may be less significant. However, even with positive pressure high-volume irrigation, head-down or lateral position may lead to better frontal distribution.[5,30]

Fluid Volume

There are limited data on the exact volume required to allow complete distribution. Higher volumes do seem to penetrate both maxillary and frontal sinus with good coverage starting at about 100 mL.[30] The frontal and sphenoid sinuses are not accessed well by pressurized spray when compared with high-volume devices such as squeeze bottles or Neti pots.[5] From current research, higher volume and positive

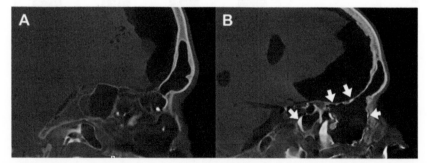

Fig. 6. Computed tomography of contrast distribution during nasal irrigation. (*A*) Before surgery; (*B*) after surgery, demonstrating the extent of fluid reached (*arrows*). A variety of other fluid dynamic factors are not recorded in this method, such as volume, force, turbulence, and shearing potential.

pressure irrigation are likely to result in the best distribution. Squeeze bottles offer one option for this approach (**Fig. 7**).

MICRODELIVERY

Significant local mucosal factors are often overlooked in establishing the effectiveness of local drug delivery. Little is still known about the mucus blanket in the airway. Much research is extrapolated from intestinal mucosal study.[31] The presence and composition of the mucus blanket, mucociliary clearance, direct mucin-drug binding, and the permeability of pharmaceutical compounds all contribute to altered drug delivery.[32] For drugs to have good bioavailability and avoid rapid clearance, they must traverse the outer layers of the mucus barrier quickly, and be adherent or rapidly permeate the epithelial surface.

Mucus Blanket

Nasal mucus is a significant barrier to airway drug delivery.[33] Nasal mucus is a powerful first line of defense for the body's airway as it copes with more than 500 liters of air that is filtered into the system per hour.[34] It is thought that more than 25 million particles are managed every hour by the airway epithelium.[35] The mucus blanket is a viscoelastic gel that forms a film over respiratory epithelium. The blanket's production is highly inducible and can increase in thickness by as much as 10 μm per second[36] on stimulation. For many inflammatory airway conditions, there is substantial mucus hypersecretion.[37–40] Hypersecretion is a similar defining feature in rhinitis[41] and CRS.[42]

Enhanced drug delivery without a mucus blanket
Removal of the mucus blanket may enhance drug absorption. There is evidence of a synergistic effect of hypertonic saline and topical steroid delivery. It is possible that removal of the mucus blanket alone may allow better steroid absorption.

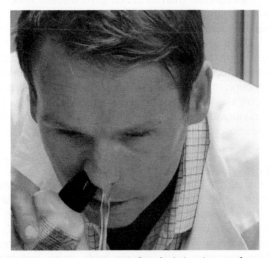

Fig. 7. High-volume positive pressure squeeze bottle irrigation performed with retrograde flow in contralateral nose after ESS offers the best fluid distribution to the sinuses from recent fluid dynamic research. (*Courtesy of* Division of Rhinology, St Vincent's Hospital; with permission.)

Alterations to tight junction permeability may also enhance drug absorption.[43] There is evidence that increased tight junction permeability of respiratory mucosa occurs with hypertonic saline and is not seen with equivalent mannitol osmolarity.[44] Whether this leads to better intranasal steroid delivery is a matter of debate. There is evidence to support a synergistic effect of saline and steroid from clinical trials in rhinitis[45,46] and from nebulized therapy in asthma.[47,48]

Mechanical removal of sinonasal secretions, antigens, or biofilm

The potential for sprays and irrigations to remove debris, mucus, or antigen has always been implied. However, there is little research to substantiate its effectiveness. There is only indirect evidence of reduced antigen-specific IgE levels in allergic rhinitis sufferers who use saline during the allergy season.[49] High-volume solutions seem to be more effective in managing CRS symptoms than simple sprays,[50] but with mixed groups of pre- and post-ESS patients the degree of benefit is still debatable. Although assumed to be effective, positive pressure irrigations may potentially seed antigens and inflammatory mucus products throughout the paranasal sinuses, as demonstrated by the positive pressure effects of nose blowing.[51]

Diffusion and permeability through the mucus blanket

Nasal mucus consists of a layered non-Newtonian shearing fluid blanket. This blanket produces a periciliary layer with watery secretions that maintains fluidity for ciliary coupling of the outer layer, commonly referred to as the gel or viscoelastic gel layer.[31] Of importance, each layer is relatively unstirred, with shearing forces between the 2 layers. Secreted surfactants are thought to concentrate in the transition zone and facilitate this process.[52] The volume and thickness is difficult to determine, as techniques for imaging the layers often add to distortion. An accepted average thickness is 15 µm,[33,53] consisting of at least 5 to 10 µm for the periciliary layer to allow immersion of the cilia. This layer combines with a gel layer of various thicknesses, 7 to 30 µm in healthy states[54,55] and greater than 50 to 200 µm is disease states.[32,56] The blanket consists of cross-linked and entangled mucin fibers secreted by goblet cells and submucosal glands.[57] Mucins are approximately 3 to 10 µm in diameter with a length of about 15 µm.[31] The mucins form a 3-dimensional web with an interfiber space ranging from 10 to 200 µm (**Fig. 8**).[33] Hydrophobic domains in mucus hinder the diffusion of many drugs. Hydrophobic compounds will often diffuse slower through mucus than water.[58,59] Although physical obstruction is presented to particulate matter, the mucin fibers are highly elastic and low-affinity interactions do allow larger macromolecules, such as immunoglobulin, to diffuse through the layers. Small neutral molecules diffuse faster, as do liposome and microsphere-bearing drugs.[60]

Mucin binding of delivered drugs

In a nondiseased state, the mucus comprises 2% proteins. Mucins are either membrane-bound or secreted, and consist of proline, threonine, or serine domains on linear peptide backbones.[61] High-density mucin glycoproteins define much of the elasticity and viscosity of airway mucus.[62] MUC5B, MUC5AC, and MUC2 are the main secreted mucins in the sinonasal tract.[34,42,63] In addition to mucin, long chains of DNA from degraded cells, organic lipids, salts, lactoferrins, lysozymes, immunoglobulins, and other proteins add to the mucus content. Little is known about mucins and other mucus-related proteins regarding their potential drug-binding ability.

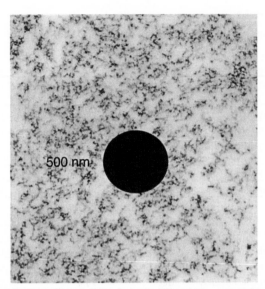

Fig. 8. The tangled mucin web that presents a mechanical barrier to larger drug particles. The intermucin channels are usually 10 to 200 μm and a 500-μm area is shown for comparison. Changes to surface chemistry can produce favorable properties that will allow larger particles to penetrate. (*From* Cone RA. Barrier properties of mucus. Adv Drug Deliv Rev 2009;61:75–85; with permission.)

Mucociliary Clearance

Sinonasal residence, or the time a formulation is in contact with its absorbing membrane, has important consequences for the bioavailability of a delivered drug. Mucociliary function propels nasal cavity mucus at a rate of 5 to 11 mm/min,[64–67] and will clear the nasal cavity in 10 minutes[67] and the maxillary sinus in 20 minutes.[68] Researchers have long being trying to improve the mucoadhesiveness of mucosally delivered drugs. Mucoadhesiveness is usually achieved by hydrogen bonding, polymer entanglements with mucins, hydrophobic domains, or a combination of these.[33]

Common polymers employed for this purpose have included carbopol, carboxymethylcellulose, polyacrylic acid, and chitin.[60] Chitosan, a cationic polymer and derivative of chitin, can improve mucoadhesion in oral and nasally delivered drugs.[69,70] Powdered delivery polymers such as carbopol can increase bioavailability of apomorphine from 45% to 98% compared with the aqueous formulation.[71] Budesonide esterification can aid entanglement with mucins and improves nasal residency, mucoadhesiveness, and bioavaliability.[72] When combined with polyethylene glycol, budesonide demonstrated longer drug release and absorption.[73] Antibiotics, such as gentamicin and ciprofloxacin, can also be delivered with mucoadherent properties. Hyaluronic acid and hyaluronic acid/chitin microspheres can enhance nasal delivery of gentamicin.[74,75] Ciprofloxacin, when combined with hydroxypropyl methylcellulose, can reach bioavailability similar to that achieved by the oral route (**Table 2**).[78] Safety concerns are not without merit, as further disruption to the mucociliary clearance or superinfection of the respiratory tract is possible.

Gravity-Affected Areas

Refractory inflammatory sinus disease is often reported in the mucosa of the ethmoid roof and frontal recess.[79,80] Is the ethmoid roof and frontal sinus an immunologically

Table 2
Examples of mucoadhesive effects on bioavailability

Drugs	Mucoadhesive Agents	Dosage Forms	Bioavailability (%)	Study
Budesonide	(P(MAA-g-EG)) microspheres	Powder	83.9	Nakamura et al[73]
Gentamicin	Hyaluronan	Powder	23.3	Lim et al[74,75]
Gentamicin	Chitosan	Powder	31.4	Lim et al[74,75]
Gentamicin	Hyaluronan/ chitosan	Powder	42.9	Lim et al[74,75]
Leuprolide	HPC/MCC	Powder	34.9	Suzuki 1999[76]
Calcitonin	HPC/MCC	Powder	16.4	Suzuki 1999[76]
Calcitonin	Chitosan free amine	Liquid	2.5	Sinswat 2003[77]
Ciprofloxacin	HPMC	Gel	40.2	Ozsoy et al[78]
Ciprofloxacin	HEC	Gel	19.5	Ozsoy et al[78]
Ciprofloxacin	MC	Gel	18.2	Ozsoy et al[78]
Ciprofloxacin	HEC + Tween 80	Gel	25.4	Ozsoy et al[78]
Ciprofloxacin	MC + Tween 80	Gel	22.3	Ozsoy et al[78]

Abbreviations: HEC, hydroxyethyl cellulose; HPC, hydroxypropyl cellulose; HPMC, hydroxypropyl-methyl cellulose; LPC, l-a-lysophosphatidylcholine; MC, methylcellulose; MCC, microcrystalline cellulose; P(MAA-g-EG), polymethacrylic acid and polyethylene glycol; rel, relative.
Data from Ugwoke MI, Agu RU, Verbeke N, et al. Nasal mucoadhesive drug delivery: background, applications, trends and future perspectives. Adv Drug Deliv Rev 2005:57;1640–65.

unique place, or are they simply poorly penetrated and have very short contact time or residency? Combined with poor distribution to these areas,[5] mucosal residence of any therapeutic agent is likely to be further reduced by gravity-dependent flow from the ethmoid roof and frontal sinus, thus making these regions poorly managed with topical therapy.

Novel Agents

Mucoactive agents: surfactants

Amphipathic molecules possess the ability to be soluble in both water and organic solutions; they form the basis of surfactants, which affect both the solution and remaining molecular load behavior at air-surface interfaces.[81] Pulmonary surfactant is the best known clinical example of these important amphipathic molecules. Pulmonary surfactant greatly improves the efficiency of mucociliary clearance by reducing adhesiveness of mucus to the respiratory epithelium. The case of acute respiratory distress of the newborn is an example of when such agents are required in normal respiratory function. Surfactants can have mucoactive and antimicrobial properties. Chemical surfactants can interfere with microbial cell membrane permeability and cause membrane disruption. These agents are often classified as cationic, anionic, or zwitterionic (possessing nonadjacent positive and negative charges) based on the charge of the hydrophilic domain present in these molecules. Cationic surfactants possess the most antimicrobial properties but are also the most irritating.[82]

There are many commercially produced surfactants. Synthetically produced detergents, soil wetting agents, paints, antifogging solutions, and ski wax are all examples. The combination of PEG-80 sorbitan laurate, cocamidopropyl betaine, and sodium trideceth sulfate (commonly known as Johnson & Johnson Baby Shampoo) has been shown to have antibiofilm-forming properties at 1% solution and clinical efficacy in managing refractory CRS patients.[82] It is currently unclear which subsets of CRS patients would benefit from such therapies.

Citric acid zwitterionic surfactant (CAZS) is currently under study for potential antimicrobial activity.[83] This agent combines the calcium bridge disrupting citric acid with the surfactant, caprylyl sulfobetaine. CAZS was effective in reducing bacterial-forming units within a sheep CRS model but not as effective as topical mupirocin.[84] There are concerns regarding possible ciliary dysfunction from any synthetic additive, and future combination solutions are likely to lead to effective agents.

Mucolytic agents may also have a role in enhancing local drug delivery.[85] Recombinant human DNase, also known as Dornase alfa, has been commonly used in the treatment of cystic fibrosis.[86,87] Dornase alfa hydrolyses the long chains of DNA that forms further entanglements in mucins. Although this has helped improve the viscoelastic properties of mucus, drug diffusion rates do not seem to be affected.[88] Other mucolytics may have a role in improving absorption. N-Acetylcysteine breaks the mucin cross-linking by cleaving disulfide bonds.[89] Mucolytics have been shown to improve the mucus diffusion for nonviral gene vectors.[90]

Second-generation mucoadhesives

Newer mucoadhesives have drug-polymer interactions that allow sustained drug release to the mucosa with less toxicity to normal sinonasal physiology. Polymers that alter their viscoelastic properties based on pH or thermal changes may provide one approach. Budesonide-linked copolymers of polymethacrylic acid and polyethylene glycol in powder form swell in response to pH changes, creating a gel, and provide a sustained release in nasal mucosa.[73] pH-sensitive chitosan[91] and polycarbophil[92] also have similar potential for nasal delivery. Thermoresponsive polymers have produced up to 11-fold increases in DNA absorption, and can be manipulated for "gelation" to occur at sinonasal temperatures.[93] Other bioadhesive activity, such as cytoadhesion, may also improve delivery. Lectin, a naturally occurring glycoprotein, can be linked to therapeutic molecules for epithelial adhesion and internalization.[94] Toxicity of these newer bioadhesives will need to be demonstrated, as they are not simply modifications of compounds already in use.

Mucopenetration

Mucoadhesion strategies that attempt to enhance local drug delivery by overcoming natural respiratory defense mechanisms will always have limitations. Mucociliary clearance, gravity-dependent drainage, mucin binding, and the perpetual turnover of mucus are normal physiologic actions that will lead to diffusion and removal of any active topical agents before these agents actually reach the respiratory epithelium or other cellular targets, thus hindering this approach. Mucus-penetrating strategies, such as nanoparticles smaller than 100 μm, will enable novel drugs to be delivered via a transmucosal route (**Fig. 9**). Alterations to surface chemistry to incorporate uncharged and hydrophilic polymers, such as polyethylene glycol (PEG), may provide a relatively mucoinert compound able to traverse the mucus blanket and be rapidly absorbed.[95] This approach improved absorption 3-fold for 100- to 500-mm particles and to a greater degree for larger molecules. Mucopenetrating, noncharged surface nanoparticles with immunogenicity similar to viral vectors may allow for an effective drug delivery system to mucosal surfaces.

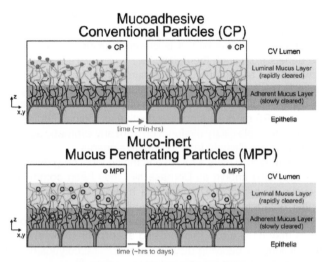

Fig. 9. The fate of mucus-penetrating particles (MPP) and conventional mucoadhesive particles (CP) administered to a mucosal surface. MPP readily penetrate the luminal mucus layer (LML) and enter the underlying adherent mucus layer (AML). In contrast, CP are largely immobilized in the LML. Because MPP can enter the AML and thus are in closer proximity to the cells, cells will be exposed to a greater dose of drug released from MPP compared with drug released from CP. As the LML layer is cleared, CP are removed along with the LML whereas MPP in the AML are retained, leading to prolonged residence time for MPP at the mucosal surface. Thus, at long times there is almost no drug dosing to cells with CP, whereas MPP, because they are retained longer, will continue to release drugs to cells. Because MPP can penetrate both the LML and AML, a fraction may reach and bind to the underlying epithelia and further improve drug delivery. Although this schematic reflects the mucosal physiology of the gastrointestinal and cervicovaginal tracts, the same behavior is expected for the respiratory airways. In the respiratory airways, CP are mostly immobilized in the luminal stirred mucus gel layer, whereas MPP penetrate the mucus gel and enter the underlying periciliary layer. On mucociliary clearance, a significant fraction of MPP remains in the periciliary layer, resulting in prolonged retention. This schematic does not depict the glycocalyx adjacent to the epithelial surface, which may contribute an additional steric barrier to cellular entry of MPP. (*From* Lai SK, Wang YY, Hanes J. Mucus-penetrating nanoparticles for drug and gene delivery to mucosal tissues. Adv Drug Deliv Rev 2009;61:158–71; with permission.)

SUMMARY

Physicians are currently faced with a bewildering array of topical therapies available for their patients with rhinosinusitis. Topical therapies will continue to grow in popularity due to their ease, efficacy, and targeted approach to the end organ in CRS, the sinonasal mucosa. There is currently little evidence to support the use of topical therapies delivered via low-volume devices, such as nebulizers or sprays, in the unoperated state. In addition, most topical therapies used before ESS do not reach the paranasal sinuses to any significant extent and are simply treating nasal conditions, such as turbinate and nasal mucosal reactivity. As the knowledge base of the precise pathophysiology of the various subsets of CRS grows, it will enable otolaryngologists to tailor topical therapies that are specific for the type of CRS seen in each patient. The pharmacologic additives used must be selected with a purpose in mind, that is, to target antimicrobials, anti-inflammatories, surfactants, or mucorheologic modulating agents. One solution will likely not be the treatment of choice for all CRS patients. Otolaryngologists must have a comprehensive understanding of topical therapies that are available, when to use specific agents, and how to deliver them, to provide maximal benefit to their patients.

REFERENCES

1. Fokkens W, Lund V, Mullol J, et al. European position paper on rhinosinusitis and nasal polyps 2007. Rhinol Suppl 2007;1–136.
2. Kern RC, Conley DB, Walsh W, et al. Perspectives on the etiology of chronic rhinosinusitis: an immune barrier hypothesis. Am J Rhinol 2008;22:549–59.
3. Lund VJ. Therapeutic targets in rhinosinusitis: infection or inflammation? Medscape J Med 2008;10:105.
4. Hatipoglu U, Rubinstein I. Anti-inflammatory treatment of chronic rhinosinusitis: a shifting paradigm. Curr Allergy Asthma Rep 2008;8:154–61.
5. Harvey RJ, Goddard JC, Wise SK, et al. Effects of endoscopic sinus surgery and delivery device on cadaver sinus irrigation. Otolaryngol Head Neck Surg 2008; 139:137–42.
6. Snidvongs K, Chaowanapanja P, Aeumjaturapat S, et al. Does nasal irrigation enter paranasal sinuses in chronic rhinosinusitis? Am J Rhinol 2008;22:483–6.
7. Hyo N, Takano H, Hyo Y. Particle deposition efficiency of therapeutic aerosols in the human maxillary sinus. Rhinology 1989;27:17–26.
8. Wormald P-J, Cain T, Oates L, et al. A comparative study of three methods of nasal irrigation. Laryngoscope 2004;114:2224–7.
9. Olson D, Rasgon B, Hilsinger R. Radiographic comparison of three methods for nasal saline irrigation. Laryngoscope 2002;112:1394–8.
10. Grobler A, Weitzel EK, Buele A, et al. Pre- and postoperative sinus penetration of nasal irrigation. Laryngoscope 2008;118:2078–81.
11. Hwang PH, Woo RJ, Fong KJ. Intranasal deposition of nebulized saline: a radionuclide distribution study. Am J Rhinol 2006;20:255–61.
12. DelGaudio JM, Wise SK. Topical steroid drops for the treatment of sinus ostia stenosis in the postoperative period. Am J Rhinol 2006;20:563–7.
13. Lavigne F, Cameron L, Renzi PM, et al. Intrasinus administration of topical budesonide to allergic patients with chronic rhinosinusitis following surgery. Laryngoscope 2002;112:858–64.
14. Mastalerz L, Milewski M, Duplaga M, et al. Intranasal fluticasone propionate for chronic eosinophilic rhinitis in patients with aspirin-induced asthma. Allergy 1997;52:895–900.
15. Qvarnberg Y, Kantola O, Salo J, et al. Influence of topical steroid treatment on maxillary sinusitis. Rhinology 1992;30:103–12.
16. Parikh A, Scadding GK, Darby Y, et al. Topical corticosteroids in chronic rhinosinusitis: a randomized, double-blind, placebo-controlled trial using fluticasone propionate aqueous nasal spray. Rhinology 2001;39:75–9.
17. Dijkstra MD, Ebbens FA, Poublon RM, et al. Fluticasone propionate aqueous nasal spray does not influence the recurrence rate of chronic rhinosinusitis and nasal polyps 1 year after functional endoscopic sinus surgery. Clin Exp Allergy 2004;34:1395–400.
18. Chiu AG, Kennedy DW. Disadvantages of minimal techniques for surgical management of chronic rhinosinusitis. Curr Opin Otolaryngol Head Neck Surg 2004;12:38–42.

19. Valentine R, Athanasiadis T, Thwin M, et al. A prospective controlled trial of pulsed nasal nebulizer in maximally dissected cadavers. Am J Rhinol 2008;22:390–4.
20. Miller TR, Muntz HR, Gilbert ME, et al. Comparison of topical medication delivery systems after sinus surgery. Laryngoscope 2004;114(2):201–4.
21. Merkus P, Ebbens FA, Muller B, et al. The 'best method' of topical nasal drug delivery: comparison of seven techniques. Rhinology 2006;44:102–7.
22. Karagama YG, Lancaster JL, Karkanevatos A, et al. Delivery of nasal drops to the middle meatus: which is the best head position? Rhinology 2001;39:226–9.
23. Kayarkar R, Clifton NJ, Woolford TJ. An evaluation of the best head position for instillation of steroid nose drops. Clin Otolaryngol Allied Sci 2002;27:18–21.
24. Homer JJ, Raine CH. An endoscopic photographic comparison of nasal drug delivery by aqueous spray. Clin Otolaryngol Allied Sci 1998;23:560–3.
25. Homer JJ, Maughan J, Burniston M. A quantitative analysis of the intranasal delivery of topical nasal drugs to the middle meatus: spray versus drop administration. J Laryngol Otol 2002;116:10–3.
26. Aggarwal R, Cardozo A, Homer JJ. The assessment of topical nasal drug distribution. Clin Otolaryngol Allied Sci 2004;29:201–5.
27. Tsikoudas A, Homer JJ. The delivery of topical nasal sprays and drops to the middle meatus: a semiquantitative analysis. Clin Otolaryngol Allied Sci 2001;26:294–7.
28. Cannady SB, Batra PS, Citardi MJ, et al. Comparison of delivery of topical medications to the paranasal sinuses via "vertex-to-floor" position and atomizer spray after FESS. Otolaryngol Head Neck Surg 2005;133:735–40.
29. Benninger MS, Hadley JA, Osguthorpe JD, et al. Techniques of intranasal steroid use. Otolaryngol Head Neck Surg 2004;130:5–24.
30. Beule A, Athanasiadis T, Athanasiadis E, et al. Efficacy of different techniques of sinonasal irrigation after modified Lothrop procedure. Am J Rhinol Allergy 2009;23:85–90.
31. Mestecky J. Mucosal immunology. In: Mestecky J, editor. 3rd edition, vol 2. Amsterdam; London: Elsevier Academic Press; 2005. p. 1868–918.
32. Widdicombe JG. Airway liquid: a barrier to drug diffusion? Eur Respir J 1997;10:2194–7.
33. Lai SK, Wang YY, Hanes J. Mucus-penetrating nanoparticles for drug and gene delivery to mucosal tissues. Adv Drug Deliv Rev 2009;61:158–71.
34. Rogers DF. Physiology of airway mucus secretion and pathophysiology of hypersecretion. Respir Care 2007;52:1134–46 [discussion 1146–9].
35. Seaton A, MacNee W, Donaldson K, et al. Particulate air pollution and acute health effects. Lancet 1995;345:176–8.
36. Rogers DF, Lethem MI. Airway mucus: basic mechanisms and clinical perspectives. Basel: Birkhauser Verlag; 1997.
37. Aikawa T, Shimura S, Sasaki H, et al. Morphometric analysis of intraluminal mucus in airways in chronic obstructive pulmonary disease. Am Rev Respir Dis 1989;140:477–82.
38. Openshaw PJ, Turner-Warwick M. Observations on sputum production in patients with variable airflow obstruction; implications for the diagnosis of asthma and chronic bronchitis. Respir Med 1989;83:25–31.
39. Rogers DF. Airway mucus hypersecretion in asthma: an undervalued pathology? Curr Opin Pharmacol 2004;4:241–50.
40. Turner-Warwick M, Openshaw P. Sputum in asthma. Postgrad Med J 1987;63(Suppl 1):79–82.
41. Martinez-Anton A, Roca-Ferrer J, Mullol J. Mucin gene expression in rhinitis syndromes. Curr Allergy Asthma Rep 2006;6:189–97.

42. Kim DH, Chu H-S, Lee JY, et al. Up-regulation of MUC5AC and MUC5B mucin genes in chronic rhinosinusitis. Arch Otolaryngol Head Neck Surg 2004;130:747–52.

43. Agu RU, Vu Dang H, Jorissen M, et al. Nasal absorption enhancement strategies for therapeutic peptides: an in vitro study using cultured human nasal epithelium. Int J Pharm 2002;237:179–91.

44. Hogman M, Mork AC, Roomans GM. Hypertonic saline increases tight junction permeability in airway epithelium. Eur Respir J 2002;20:1444–8.

45. Slapak I, Skoupa J, Strnad P, et al. Efficacy of isotonic nasal wash (seawater) in the treatment and prevention of rhinitis in children. Arch Otolaryngol Head Neck Surg 2008;134:67–74.

46. Harvey R, Hannan SA, Badia L, et al. Nasal saline irrigations for the symptoms of chronic rhinosinusitis. Cochrane Database Syst Rev 2007;3:CD006394.

47. Rogers DF. Mucoactive agents for airway mucus hypersecretory diseases. Respir Care 2007;52:1176–93 [discussion 1193–77].

48. Daviskas E, Anderson SD. Hyperosmolar agents and clearance of mucus in the diseased airway. J Aerosol Med 2006;19:100–9.

49. Subiza JL, Subiza J, Barjau MC, et al. Inhibition of the seasonal IgE increase to *Dactylis glomerata* by daily sodium chloride nasal-sinus irrigation during the grass pollen season. J Allergy Clin Immunol 1999;104:711–2.

50. Pynnonen MA, Mukerji SS, Kim HM, et al. Nasal saline for chronic sinonasal symptons: a randomized controlled trail. Archi Otolaryngol—Head Neck Surg 2007;133:1115–20.

51. Gwaltney JM Jr, Hendley JO, Phillips CD, et al. Nose blowing propels nasal fluid into the paranasal sinuses. Clin Infect Dis 2000;30:387–91.

52. Morgenroth K, Bolz J. Morphological features of the interaction between mucus and surfactant on the bronchial mucosa. Respiration 1985;47:225–31.

53. Sleigh MA, Blake JR, Liron N. The propulsion of mucus by cilia. Am Rev Respir Dis 1988;137:726–41.

54. Matsui H, Grubb BR, Tarran R, et al. Evidence for periciliary liquid layer depletion, not abnormal ion composition, in the pathogenesis of cystic fibrosis airways disease. Cell 1998;95:1005–15.

55. Tarran R, Grubb BR, Gatzy JT, et al. The relative roles of passive surface forces and active ion transport in the modulation of airway surface liquid volume and composition. J Gen Physiol 2001;118:223–36.

56. Widdicombe J. Airway and alveolar permeability and surface liquid thickness: theory. J Appl Physiol 1997;82:3–12.

57. Thornton DJ, Sheehan JK. From mucins to mucus: toward a more coherent understanding of this essential barrier. Proc Am Thorac Soc 2004;1:54–61.

58. Khanvilkar K, Donovan MD, Flanagan DR. Drug transfer through mucus. Adv Drug Deliv Rev 2001;48:173–93.

59. Larhed AW, Artursson P, Grasjo J, et al. Diffusion of drugs in native and purified gastrointestinal mucus. J Pharm Sci 1997;86:660–5.

60. Ugwoke MI, Agu RU, Verbeke N, et al. Nasal mucoadhesive drug delivery: background, applications, trends and future perspectives. Adv Drug Deliv Rev 2005;57:1640–65.

61. Rose MC, Voynow JA. Respiratory tract mucin genes and mucin glycoproteins in health and disease. Physiol Rev 2006;86:245–78.

62. Rubin BK. Physiology of airway mucus clearance. Respir Care 2002;47:761–8.

63. Pena MT, Aujla PK, Patel KM, et al. Immunohistochemical analyses of MUC5AC mucin expression in sinus mucosa of children with sinusitis and controls. Ann Otol Rhinol Laryngol 2005;114:958–65.

64. Proctor DF. The upper airways. I. Nasal physiology and defense of the lungs. Am Rev Respir Dis 1977;115:97–129.
65. Illum L. Nasal drug delivery—possibilities, problems and solutions. J Control Release 2003;87:187–98.
66. Saketkhoo K, Januszkiewicz A, Sackner MA. Effects of drinking hot water, cold water, and chicken soup on nasal mucus velocity and nasal airflow resistance. Chest 1978;74:408–10.
67. Schuhl JF. Nasal mucociliary clearance in perennial rhinitis. J Investig Allergol Clin Immunol 1995;5:333–6.
68. Ali MS, Pearson JP. Upper airway mucin gene expression: a review. Laryngoscope 2007;117:932–8.
69. Bernkop-Schnurch A. Thiomers: a new generation of mucoadhesive polymers. Adv Drug Deliv Rev 2005;57:1569–82.
70. Prego C, Torres D, Alonso MJ. The potential of chitosan for the oral administration of peptides. Expert Opin Drug Deliv 2005;2:843–54.
71. Sam E, Jeanjean AP, Maloteaux JM, et al. Apomorphine pharmacokinetics in parkinsonism after intranasal and subcutaneous application. Eur J Drug Metab Pharmacokinet 1995;20:27–33.
72. Petersen H, Kullberg A, Edsbacker S, et al. Nasal retention of budesonide and fluticasone in man: formation of airway mucosal budesonide-esters in vivo. Br J Clin Pharmacol 2001;51:159–63.
73. Nakamura K, Maitani Y, Lowman AM, et al. Uptake and release of budesonide from mucoadhesive, pH-sensitive copolymers and their application to nasal delivery. J Control Release 1999;61:329–35.
74. Lim ST, Martin GP, Berry DJ, et al. Preparation and evaluation of the in vitro drug release properties and mucoadhesion of novel microspheres of hyaluronic acid and chitosan. J Control Release 2000;66:281–92.
75. Lim ST, Forbes B, Martin GP, et al. In vivo and in vitro characterization of novel microparticulates based on hyaluronan and chitosan hydroglutamate. AAPS PharmSciTech 2001;2:20.
76. Suzuki Y, Makino Y. Mucosal drug delivery using cellulose derivatives as a functional polymer. J Control Release 1999;62:101–7.
77. Sinswat P, Tengamnuary P. Enhancing effect of chitosan on nasal absorption of salman calcitonin in rats: comparison with hydroxypropyl- and dimethyl-beta-cyclodextrins. Int J Phamaceutics 2003;257:15–22.
78. Ozsoy Y, Tuncel T, Can A, et al. In vivo studies on nasal preparations of ciprofloxacin hydrochloride. Pharmazie 2000;55:607–9.
79. Desrosiers M. Refractory chronic rhinosinusitis: pathophysiology and management of chronic rhinosinusitis persisting after endoscopic sinus surgery. Curr Allergy Asthma Rep 2004;4:200–7.
80. Citardi MJ, Kuhn FA. Endoscopically guided frontal sinus beclomethasone instillation for refractory frontal sinus/recess mucosal edema and polyposis. Am J Rhinol 1998;12:179–82.
81. Van Hamme JD, Singh A, Ward OP. Physiological aspects. Part 1 in a series of papers devoted to surfactants in microbiology and biotechnology. Biotechnol Adv 2006;24:604–20.
82. Chiu AG, Palmer JN, Woodworth BA, et al. Baby shampoo nasal irrigations for the symptomatic postfunctional endoscopic sinus surgery patient. Am J Rhinol 2008;22:34–7.
83. Desrosiers M, Myntti M, James G. Methods for removing bacterial biofilms: in vitro study using clinical chronic rhinosinusitis specimens. Am J Rhinol 2007;21:527–32.

84. Le T, Psaltis A, Tan LW, et al. The efficacy of topical antibiofilm agents in a sheep model of rhinosinusitis. Am J Rhinol 2008;22:560–7.
85. Lai SK, Wang YY, Wirtz D, et al. Micro- and macrorheology of mucus. Adv Drug Deliv Rev 2009;61:86–100.
86. Shah PL, Scott SF, Knight RA, et al. In vivo effects of recombinant human DNase I on sputum in patients with cystic fibrosis. Thorax 1996;51:119–25.
87. Cimmino M, Nardone M, Cavaliere M, et al. Dornase alfa as postoperative therapy in cystic fibrosis sinonasal disease. Arch Otolaryngol Head Neck Surg 2005;131:1097–101.
88. Dawson M, Wirtz D, Hanes J. Enhanced viscoelasticity of human cystic fibrotic sputum correlates with increasing microheterogeneity in particle transport. J Biol Chem 2003;278:50393–401.
89. Henke MO, Ratjen F. Mucolytics in cystic fibrosis. Paediatr Respir Rev 2007;8: 24–9.
90. Ferrari S, Kitson C, Farley R, et al. Mucus altering agents as adjuncts for nonviral gene transfer to airway epithelium. Gene Ther 2001;8:1380–6.
91. Hornof MD, Kast CE, Bernkop-Schnurch A. In vitro evaluation of the viscoelastic properties of chitosan-thioglycolic acid conjugates. Eur J Pharm Biopharm 2003; 55:185–90.
92. Bernkop-Schnurch A, Scholler S, Biebel RG. Development of controlled drug release systems based on thiolated polymers. J Control Release 2000;66:39–48.
93. Park JS, Oh YK, Yoon H, et al. In situ gelling and mucoadhesive polymer vehicles for controlled intranasal delivery of plasmid DNA. J Biomed Mater Res 2002;59: 144–51.
94. Lehr CM. Lectin-mediated drug delivery: the second generation of bioadhesives. J Control Release 2000;65:19–29.
95. Lai SK, O'Hanlon DE, Harrold S, et al. Rapid transport of large polymeric nano-particles in fresh undiluted human mucus. Proc Natl Acad Sci U S A 2007;104: 1482–7.

Balloon Dilatation of the Paranasal Sinuses: A Tool in Sinus Surgery

Esther Kim, MD[a], Jeffrey L. Cutler, MD[a,b],*

KEYWORDS

- Balloon sinuplasty • Balloon catheter ostial dilatation
- Chronic rhinosinusitis • Minimally invasive sinus surgery
- Office sinus surgery

Close to 31 million Americans suffer from chronic rhinosinusitis.[1] Endoscopic sinus surgery is currently the mainstay of treatment of patients who have failed medical management. The goals of surgery, traditionally, have been to remove inflamed tissue and bone to improve ventilation and drainage of the affected sinuses. Like all aspects of surgery, sinus surgery has evolved greatly since its inception.

Over the years, several notable pioneers have changed the way in which sinonasal disorders are treated. Near the turn of the nineteenth century, George Caldwell and Henri Luc individually described the canine fossa approach to the maxillary sinus. Nasal endoscopy was first used in 1901 by Hirshman, using a modified cystoscope.[2] The development of the Hopkins rod telescope, patented in 1960, further revolutionized sinus surgery and enabled the otolaryngologist to navigate through the nasal cavity with unparalleled visualization. In 1978, Messerklinger[3] published a collection of images detailing his surgical experience, which is considered a landmark in endoscopic sinus surgery. In the mid-1980s, Stammberger[4–6] published a series of papers describing endoscopic sinus surgery techniques. Kennedy and colleagues[7] brought these innovative techniques to the United States and coined the term "functional endoscopic sinus surgery."

Image guidance systems, which were originally developed for neurosurgeons, have transitioned well into the operating room for sinus surgeons. The utility of this technology has allowed sinus surgeons to stretch the boundaries of endonasal procedures to include treatment of anterior skull base lesions. Although the use of image guidance

Jeffrey L. Cutler, MD is a consultant, stockholder, and serves on the Scientific Advisory Board for Entellus Medical, Inc.

[a] Department of Surgery, Section of Otolaryngology, Head and Neck Surgery, Walter Reed Army Medical Center, 6900 Georgia Avenue, NW, Washington, DC 20307, USA

[b] Uniform Services University of the Health Sciences, NW, Washington, DC

* Corresponding author. Department of Surgery, Section of Otolaryngology, Head and Neck Surgery, Walter Reed Army Medical Center, NW, Washington, DC 20307.

E-mail address: Jeffrey.cutler@hotmail.com (J.L. Cutler).

Otolaryngol Clin N Am 42 (2009) 847–856

doi:10.1016/j.otc.2009.07.006

0030-6665/09/$ – see front matter. Published by Elsevier Inc.

oto.theclinics.com

originally met with some skepticism, many otolaryngologists have adopted this technology into their sinus surgery practice.

Balloon catheters have become available in endoscopic sinus surgery and are now a new tool to achieve the goals of sinus ostial dilatation. Balloon technology has been available for some time in other specialties, such as interventional cardiology, gastroenterology, endovascular surgery, and urology. In many instances, balloon technology has drastically changed treatment algorithms. An example of this paradigm shift is how angioplasty has now become an effective alternative to open cardiac surgery for selected patients with coronary artery disease.

Balloon catheter–based technology is a novel tool to access and dilate selected sinus ostia in patients with chronic rhinosinusitis, with the goal of preserving the mucosa and the surrounding structures. As with any new technology, there is always some degree of skepticism and doubt. In this article, the authors report on the available technology and discuss how these tools may be applied in sinus surgery. Safety and efficacy is analyzed through a review of published data.

DISCUSSION

Three companies that manufacture balloon catheters have reported their use in endoscopic sinus surgery: Acclarent, Inc (Menlo Park, CA, USA), Quest Medical, Inc (Allen, TX, USA), and Entellus Medical, Inc (Maple Grove, MN, USA). Each company is described in the following sections, including relevant published literature. Some special considerations and potential points of controversy expand the descriptions.

Acclarent, Inc

Acclarent started their first investigation of balloon catheters in 2002. Since gaining approval to use these medical devices, approximately 3000 physicians have undergone training at various training facilities. More than 20,000 patients have been treated worldwide with balloon sinuplasty.[8]

The technique involves a typical setup for endoscopic sinus surgery using a video tower and endoscopes. A guide catheter is positioned near the natural ostia of the sinus being treated. A wire is then passed through the guide catheter and is manipulated until it is confirmed to be located in the sinus cavity. The balloon catheter (**Fig. 1**) is then passed over the guide wire through the guide sheath. **Fig. 2** depicts the Acclarent Relieva system, with an endoscope and camera in a ghosted background.[9] After conformation of the appropriate location, the balloon is then inflated and released. The balloon catheters are designed for multiple sinus use in a single patient. The surgery is often performed using fluoroscopic confirmation for wire and balloon placement, but recently a lighted guide wire called Luma (**Fig. 3**) has been released. This lighted guide wire can provide a nonfluoroscopic option because direct sinus illumination can confirm location.[10] The balloon catheter dilatation can be performed on the frontal, sphenoid, and maxillary sinus outflow tracts. If needed, a traditional endoscopic ethmoidectomy can be performed in addition to balloon ostial dilatation.

An initial feasibility study was performed by Bolger and Vaughan[11] on human cadavers, with 100% success in dilating all of the 12 sinus ostia. Computed tomography (CT) scans were performed after the procedures, revealing microfractures of

Fig. 1. Acclarent Relieva Solo Pro Sinus Balloon Catheter. (*Courtesy of* Acclarent, Inc, Menlo Park, CA.)

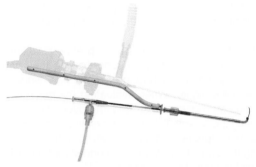

Fig. 2. Acclarent Relieva Balloon Sinuplasty System. (*Courtesy of* Acclarent, Inc, Menlo Park, CA.)

the sinus ostial regions without evidence of damage to the surrounding structure, such as the orbit or anterior skull base. This study was then followed by a pilot human study in 10 patients. Brown and Bolger[9] dilated all planned ostia and observed ease with the frontal and sphenoid sinuses; the anesthesia time was also reduced. Some difficulty was reported while dilating the maxillary sinus and removing the lower portion of the uncinate in 5 of the 10 patients. The investigators did not report any adverse events or episodes of mucosal stripping.

The publication of the results of the CLEAR study (CLinical Evaluation to confirm sAfety and efficacy of sinuplasty in the paRanasal sinuses) has been instrumental in demonstrating clinical results of balloon sinuplasty.[12–14] The study was published in 3 parts, starting with 24-week data, followed by 1-year data and then by 2-year data. The study, conducted at several institutions, comprised 115 patients. The study did not compare traditional sinus surgery with balloon sinuplasty, but evaluated hybrid procedures (balloon sinuplasty with traditional endoscopic sinus surgery, ie, ethmoidectomy) and balloon sinuplasty alone. No adverse events, including cerebral spinal fluid (CSF) leak, orbital injury, or nasal bleeding requiring nasal packing, were reported.[12–14]

The CLEAR study measured sinus symptoms using Piccirillo's validated SNOT-20 (Sino-Nasal Outcome Test) survey, which was given to the patients preoperatively and then postoperatively at 24 weeks, 1 year, and 2 years. All reports revealed a statistically significant improvement in the SNOT-20 scores. In the 2-year study, matched-pairs differences of the SNOT-20 scores were performed, and the investigators did not find any statistical difference between the scores at 24 weeks and 2 years. Similarly, there was no difference at 1 year compared with 2 years. This trend demonstrated that

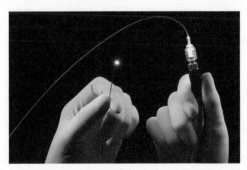

Fig. 3. Acclarent Relieva Luma Sinus Illumination System. (*Courtesy of* Acclarent, Inc, Menlo Park, CA.)

the patient's symptoms did not worsen or improve further with time after 24 weeks. The greatest improvement in the SNOT-20 survey was a reduction in facial pain and pressure.[12–14]

Another endpoint of the study was to compare preoperative and postoperative CT scans of the sinuses. The CT scans were scored using the Lund-Mackay scoring system. Patients undergoing the hybrid procedure had worse disease, and the Lund-Mackay scores were higher. When evaluating the mean for all patients in the study, the 1- and 2-year studies demonstrated improvement in Lund-Mackay scores. The difference between the scores at 1 and 2 years was not significant, indicating that there was neither further improvement nor worsening of the sinus disease as seen on CT scans. Regarding the subsets, patients who underwent the hybrid procedure had the most improvement in Lund-Mackay scores.[13,14]

A clinical outcome of the study evaluated the ostial patency during postoperative nasal endoscopy. The overall observable patency rate was 80.5% and 85% at 24 weeks and 1 year, respectively. Patency was indeterminate in 17.9% (24 weeks) and 14% (1 year) of the patients. The overall nonpatency rate was low at 1.6% at 24 weeks and 1% at 1 year. The revision rate per sinus was 0.98%, 2%, and 3.6% at 24 weeks, 1 year, and 2 years, respectively. The revision rate per patient was 2.75% and 9.2% at 24 weeks and 2 years, respectively. A functional patency rate of 91.6% was reported when a clear sinus CT scan was observed, demonstrating a functionally patent sinus ostium.[13,14]

The main criticism for the CLEAR study is the lack of randomization and the lack of a control arm. The best level of evidence as defined by the Oxford Centre for Evidence-Based Medicine is a randomized controlled clinical trial.[15] This is not always possible, and much research in sinus surgery is level IV evidence (a case series without an internal control group).[13] In addition, the investigators recognized that the improved outcomes may be influenced by a placebo effect and the natural history of the disease.[14]

The PatiENT Registry provided results of a database of a retrospective review of 1036 patients who had 3276 sinuses treated. Although the study provides level IV evidence, it does reinforce a favorable device-safety profile. The database documented only 2 CSF leaks and 6 cases of minor bleeding that required cautery or packing. These 8 cases were performed in conjunction with standard *functional endoscopic sinus surgery*. The study did illustrate a practice trend of less debridements postoperatively in sinuplasty cases. A similar revision rate to the CLEAR study was reported in that 2.4% patients underwent revision surgery.[16]

Although the CLEAR study did not report injuries to the skull base or the orbit, the MAUDE (Manufacturer and User Facility Device Experience) database reveals 5 incidents. Two reports involved penetration of the lamina papyracea, and one involved a skull base defect in a hybrid case resulting in a CSF leak. The remaining 2 cases reported balloon failure, in that the balloon broke away from the catheter.[17]

Radiation exposure

Radiation exposure with the use of fluoroscopy can be a concern to the patient and the surgeon. Radiation to the eyes can cause damage to the proliferating cells in the epithelium, and the ultimate damage is cataract formation.[18] The International Commission on Radiological Protection has stated that acute doses of 2 Gy, protracted occupational exposure of 4 Gy over less than 3 months, or 5.5 Gy over more than 3 months may cause cataract formation.[19,20] It has also been reported that an average of 4.2 mGy per eye in balloon sinuplasty, which is much less than the cataract threshold. A CT scan of the sinuses in the axial plane has an average of 24.5 mGy to the lens, and in the coronal plane it is 35.2 mGy.[21]

The surgeon is also exposed to radiation during balloon dilatation of the sinus ostia using Acclarent's system. The fluoroscope used by a surgeon for balloon sinuplasty is in direct line of the fluoroscopy tube. In comparison, the hands of the interventional cardiologist is away from the actual field of the direct "beam" while working lower near the area of the femoral vein.[8] Church studied the radiation exposure to a surgeon's hands, neck, and eyes. Using the guidelines set by the US Code of Federal Regulations, he reported that a surgeon could perform more than 57,000 dilations per year before reaching an occupational limit for the hands, 20,000 dilations per year for the neck (thyroid), and 6000 dilations per year for the eyes.[19,22,23] The direction of the fluoroscopic projection is an important factor. In the anteroposterior projection, the surgeon could perform 141 cases in a year before meeting the occupational limit for the hands.

Radiation exposure is an added risk to the patient and the surgeon. Ways to improve exposure include limiting the time of exposure by placing the fluoroscope on pulse as opposed to a continuous setting, projecting in a posteroanterior direction, shielding the patient's eyes, and protecting the operating room staff with lead aprons and thyroid shields. The use of a thyroid shield would reduce the radiation dose by up to 95%.[19] To address the radiation concern, a lighted guide wire (Luma) that can replace the need for fluoroscopy has been introduced. Direct sinus illumination by the guide wire can confirm proper location before balloon inflation.

Quest Medical, Inc

Quest Medical, Inc manufactures LacriCATH. Ophthalmologists have been using this technology to treat nasolacrimal duct obstruction since 1989. It was developed as an alternative to the open approach in treating nasolacrimal duct obstruction. The catheters have been described in an offlabel use for the treatment of sinus ostial obstruction. The catheters are unique in that they are balloons at the end of a malleable wire. This system does not require a guide wire and is available in a variety of diameters and lengths.

Citardi and Kanowitz[24] first described the use of LacriCATH in the paranasal sinuses. A cadaveric study was performed without the use of fluoroscopy. It was reported that the catheter would fracture the free wall of the frontal recess, depending on the position of the agger nasi, and the fractured bone pieces could be retrieved. In the maxillary sinus, dilatation was successfully achieved in 3 of 6 maxillaries using a prebent 9-mm balloon designed for transnasal dacryocystorhinostomy. This study demonstrated the use of existing technology to perform the task of dilating sinus ostia without the use of fluoroscopy.

A second study was performed describing the use of the LacriCATH in the office setting for revision frontal sinus stenosis. Successful dilatation of 6 frontal sinus ostia was reported in the office setting without the use of fluoroscopy. This study reviewed 6 patients only but concluded that the technique was a feasible option for the office treatment of frontal sinus stenosis.[25]

Entellus Medical, Inc

Some studies using balloon technology reported variable success in treating the maxillary sinus. Reports of trauma to adjacent structures and difficulty in identifying the natural ostium of the maxillary sinus were noted. Dilatation of the accessory ostium has also been reported. Citardi and Kanowitz[24] reported successful dilatation of the maxillary ostium using LacriCATH in only 3 of 6 sinuses. Part of this challenge is because of the difficulty in identifying the natural ostium and the tendency of the balloon to drift posteriorly through either an accessory ostium or through a posterior fontanelle.

The Entellus Medical, Inc FinESS (Functional Infundibular Endoscopic Sinus surgery) system attempts to solve this problem by direct access into the maxillary sinus through a controlled canine fossa puncture with a small trocar. An access sheath is left in place after the trocar is removed. A canula is inserted through the access sheath, through which a small endoscope and a balloon catheter can be simultaneously placed. Direct visualization with a 0.5-mm flexible endoscope (Karl Storz, El Segundo, CA, USA) (**Fig. 4**) into the maxillary sinus is performed for the identification of the natural maxillary ostium. A balloon catheter is then introduced under direct visualization through the natural ostium of the maxillary sinus and traversing the ethmoid infundibular space. The balloon is then inflated, widening the natural ostium and infundibulum and also deflecting the uncinate process medially. The maxillary sinus can then be irrigated as needed, through the canine fossa introducer. **Fig. 5** depicts the basic setup for the Entellus FinESS system.

Thirty patients were treated at 3 centers, and the results have been reported in the BREATHE I (Balloon Remodeling Antrostomy Therapy I) study.[26] Among the 58 maxillary sinus outflow tracts, 55 were effectively identified, accessed, and treated with this tool. Patient selection included individuals with chronic sinusitis affecting maxillary or the maxillary plus anterior ethmoid air cells. In addition to procedural success, safety with balloon dilatation of the maxillary sinus and ethmoid infundibulum was assessed. Patients were followed postoperatively at 1 week, 3 months, and 6 months. SNOT-20 scores were obtained at each of the follow-up visits, and a CT scan was performed at 3 months to assess ostial patency. There was a statistically significant improvement in SNOT-20 scores from baseline through the entire follow-up, and the mean scores decreased from 2.9 ± 1 to 0.8 ± 0.9 at 6 months. There were no device-related serious adverse events or unanticipated adverse device effects. CT scan volumetric analysis of the ethmoid infundibular space revealed a larger outflow tract on postoperative CT scans.[10] There were 2 reports of tooth numbness, in which 1 resolved, and 1 report of facial numbness. About 97% of the procedures were completed under local anesthesia with or without minimal intravenous sedation.

SPECIAL CONSIDERATIONS
Pain

Balloon dilatation is well tolerated by most patients. Narcotic pain medication was rarely needed as reported in the BREATHE I trial.[12] Friedman and colleagues[10] compared unmatched patients undergoing traditional endoscopic sinus surgery

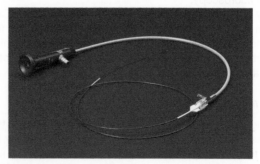

Fig. 4. Karl Storz 0.5-mm flexible endoscope. (*Courtesy of* Entellus Medical, Inc, Maple Grove, MN; with permission.)

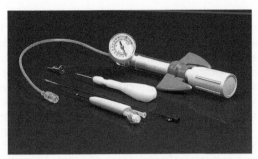

Fig. 5. Entellus FinESS balloon catheter system. (*Courtesy of* Entellus Medical, Inc, Maple Grove, MN; with permission.)

with balloon dilatation surgical candidates, and they reported less narcotic pain medication with balloon dilatation (1.34 days vs 0.8 days, $P = .011$). Patients who have undergone balloon dilatation also required much less postoperative debridement, thereby decreasing the pain from office debridement.

Cost

The average sinus surgery in the operating room involves many variables. There are disposable components and fixed costs. Geographic and institutional costs vary widely along with reimbursement. Costs of disposable components do affect the bottom line of the surgical center or hospital. Most components of all of the products described are disposable and costs can vary widely within a system. The potential shorter operative time can likely decrease the overall costs of the surgery. Friedman and colleagues did not show a significant difference in cost when comparing primary surgery performed by balloon dilatation with endoscopic sinus surgery ($14,021 vs $13,574, $P = .55$). They did show a cost benefit to balloon dilation in revision sinus surgery ($10,346 vs $16,190, $P<.0001$).[10] Despite this study, usage of these tools has been influenced by cost. However, as further research is performed and familiarity with the technology increases, the cost of the tools and the reimbursement patterns may change.

Osteitis Controversy

Surgical removal of the diseased mucosa and bone has been one of the principles of traditional sinus surgery. Clinical research has supported the importance of removal of the diseased tissue. Melroy[27] and Lanza and Kennedy[28] commented that balloon sinuplasty does not remove the diseased bone that contributes to sinusitis.[29] There are data to suggest that inflamed tissue and bone appear to potentiate the inflammatory process.[30] Staining of the bone removed by sinus surgery has shown that a remodeling occurs in the setting of chronic rhinosinusitis.[22] Thus, there are several opinions that criticize balloon technology because it does not remove the diseased tissue. Bone that has underlying osteitis may not remodel as intended by the balloon catheter. Despite this concern, it is important to realize that balloons are tools and are intended for the specific purpose of widening an outflow tract to allow ventilation and drainage. Depending on the severity of the sinus disease, the tissue may or may not need to be removed. In these circumstances, balloon dilatation with any of the choices discussed earlier may allow the surgeons to achieve their surgical goals.

Office Use

Balloon catheter ostial dilatation is a technology that seems to have the potential for office use. All 3 systems have been shown to have great promise for office-based treatment. The ability to offer local anesthesia with minimal to no sedation allows adequate patient comfort while ostial dilatation can be achieved. Recovery time is also quicker, as general anesthesia is avoided. The total cost is reduced because facility and anesthesia fees are avoided, and patients are able to quickly return to their pretreatment activities. Despite this obvious benefit in total cost reduction, wide acceptance of office use will be delayed until physician reimbursement for these office procedures is altered to account for the use of these disposable tools.

The frontal sinus can be challenging for many sinus surgeons, and postoperative stenosis can be a difficult problem. In the office, the sinus surgeon can anesthetize the patient topically, and by using a lighted guide wire for visual conformation (Acclarent) can pass a balloon catheter for frontal recess dilatation. Alternatively, if the stenotic frontal recess is well visualized, a balloon catheter on a malleable wire (LacriCATH) can be used for safe frontal recess dilatation. Luong and colleagues[22] and Citardi and Kanowitz[24] demonstrated the ease with which patients with this condition can be treated in the office. The evidence suggests that balloon catheters can be an important tool for the office management of frontal recess or ostium stenosis and can potentially avoid revision sinus surgery in the operating room.[25] Similarly, the maxillary sinus using the Entellus Medical, Inc system is well suited for office treatment. The BREATHE I results support the use of this tool under local anesthesia, as patient tolerance and satisfaction has been high.[26]

SUMMARY

Balloon catheter ostial dilatation is proving to be a useful tool to treat patients with chronic rhinosinusitis. These devices are tools to achieve the goal of ostial dilatation to allow improved ventilation and sinus drainage. Balloon catheter ostial dilatation does not replace conventional endoscopic sinus surgery but is a safe and effective tool to treat selected patients. Balloon dilatation of the sinus ostia has been shown to be safe, as all 3 manufacturers reveal a very low complication rate. Further study will help identify the sinus disease types and severity that are best addressed with these tools.

In theory, balloons may be best used in early disease states, before significant mucosal and bony osteitis has occurred. The frontal sinus can be very difficult to treat, and a balloon catheter can be an excellent dissecting tool to allow a minimal-touch technique in the right hands. Difficult and obstructing frontal cells, agger nasi cells, suprabullar ethmoid cells, and supraorbital cells can be carefully dissected with the assistance of a balloon catheter. New theories on mucosal and uncinate preservation are currently being evaluated, as the results from balloon sinus ostial dilatation appear to be providing sustainable results, although long-term follow-up is required. Advancement with these tools, with the inclusion of illuminated guide wires, direct visualization, and potential image guidance, are expanding their role in the treatment of sinus disease and are currently at the forefront of evolving sinus technology.

REFERENCES

1. Friedman M, Schalch P. Functional endoscopic dilatation of the sinuses (FEDS): patient selection and surgical technique. Operat Tech Otolaryngol Head Neck Surg 2006;17:126–34.
2. Hulett KJ, Stankiezicz AJ. "Primary sinus surgery". In: Cummings Charles, Haughey B, Thomas JRegan, et al, editors. Cummings otolaryngology: head & neck surgery. 4th edition. Philadelphia: Mosby; 2005.
3. Messerklinger W. Endoscopy of the nose. Baltimore (MD): Urban & Schwarzenberg; 1978.

4. Stammberger H. Nasal and paranasal sinus endoscopy: a diagnostic and surgical approach to recurrent sinusitis. Endoscopy 1986;18(6):213–8.
5. Stammberger H. Endoscopic endonasal surgery—concepts in treatment of recurring rhinosinusitis. Part I: anatomic and pathophysiologic considerations. Otolaryngol Head Neck Surg 1986;94(2):143–7.
6. Stammberger H. Endoscopic endonasal surgery—concepts in treatment of recurring rhinosinusitis. Part II: surgical technique. Otolaryngol Head Neck Surg 1986; 94(2):147–56.
7. Kennedy DW, Zinrich SJ, Rosenbaum AE, et al. Functional endoscopic sinus surgery. Theory and diagnostic evaluation. Arch Otolaryngol 1985;111(9):576–82.
8. Siow JK, Kadah BA, Werner AJ. Balloon sinuplasty: a current hot topic in rhinology. Eur Arch Otorhinolaryngol 2008;265:509–11.
9. Brown CL, Bolger WE. Safety and feasibility of balloon catheter dilation of paranasal sinus ostia: a preliminary investigation. Ann Otol Rhinol Laryngol 2006;115(4):293–9.
10. Friedman A, Schalch P, Lin SC, et al. Functional endoscopic dilatation of the sinuses: patient satisfaction, postoperative pain, and cost. Am J Rhinol 2008; 22:204–9.
11. Bolger WE, Vaughan W. Catheter based dilation of the sinus ostia: initial safety and feasibility in a cadaver model. Am J Rhinol 2006;20(6):290–4.
12. Bolger WE, Brown CL, Church CA, et al. Safety and outcomes of balloon catheter sinusotomy: a multicenter 24-week analysis in 115 patients. Otolaryngol Head Neck Surg 2007;137:10–20.
13. Kuhn FA, Church CA, Goldberg AN, et al. Balloon catheter sinusotomy: one-year follow-up—outcomes and role in functional endoscopic sinus surgery. Oto laryngol Head Neck Surg 2008;139:S27–37.
14. Weiss RL, Church CA, Kuhn FA, et al. Long-term analysis of balloon catheter sinusotomy: two-year follow-up. Otolaryngol Head Neck Surg 2008;138:S38–46.
15. Oxford Centre for Evidence-based Medicine - Levels of Evidence. March 2009. Available at: http://www.cebm.net/index.aspx?o=1025. Accessed June 5, 2009.
16. Levine H, Sertich AP, Hoisington DR, et al. Multicenter registry of balloon catheter sinusotomy outcomes for 1036 patients. Ann Otol Rhinol Laryngol 2008;117(4): 265–70.
17. FDA Maude Data base. April 30, 2009. Available at: http://www.accessdata.fda. gov/scripts/cdrh/cfdocs/cfMAUDE/Detail.CFM. Accessed May 27, 2009.
18. Ilgit ET, Meric N, Bor D, et al. Lens of the eye: radiation dose in balloon dacryocystoplasty. Radiology 2000;217:54–7.
19. Church CA, Kuhn FA, Mikhail J, et al. Patient and surgeon radiation exposure in balloon catheter sinus ostial dilation. Otolaryngol Head Neck Surg 2008;138:187–91.
20. Vaughan WC. Review of balloon sinuplasty. Curr Opin Otolaryngol Head Neck Surg 2008;16:2–9.
21. Zammit-Maempel I, Chadwick CL, Willis SP. Radiation dose to the lens of eye and thyroid gland in paranasal sinus multislice CT. Br J Radiol 2003;76:418–20.
22. Luong A, Batra PS, Fakhri S, et al. Balloon catheter dilatation for frontal sinus ostium stenosis in the office setting. Am J Rhinol 2008;22:621–4.
23. US Nuclear Regulatory Commission. Instruction concerning risks from occupational radiation exposure regulatory guide 8.29. February 1996. Available at: http://www.nrc.gov/reading-rm/doc-collections/reg-guides/occupational-health/ active/8-29/08-029.pdf. Accessed May 29, 2009.
24. Citardi MJ, Kanowitz SJ. A cadaveric model for balloon-assisted endoscopic paranasal sinus dissection without fluoroscopy. Am J Rhinol 2007;21:579–83.

25. Atkins J. Mechanisms of action for balloon dilation of the ostiomeatal unit in patients with chronic rhinosinusitis. Oral presentation. Rhinology World. April 17, 2009.
26. Stankiewicz J, Tami T, Truitt T, et al. Transantral, endoscopically guided balloon dilatation of the ostiomeatal complex for chronic rhinosinusitis under local anesthesia. Am J Rhinol Allergy 2009;23:1–7.
27. Melroy CT. The balloon dilating catheter as an instrument in sinus surgery. Otolaryngol Head Neck Surg 2008;139:S23–6.
28. Lanza DC, Kennedy DW. Balloon sinuplasty: not ready for prime time [commentary]. Ann Otol Rhinol Laryngol 2006;115(10):789–90.
29. Perloff JR, Gannon FH, Bolger WE, et al. Bone involvement in sinusitis: an apparent pathway for the spread of disease. Laryngoscope 2000;110:2095–9.
30. Lee JT, Kennedy DW, Palmer JN, et al. The incidence of concurrent osteitis in patients with chronic rhinosinusitis: a clinicopathological study. Am J Rhinol 2006;20(3):278–82.

Stents and Drug-Eluting Stents

Karen A. Bednarski, MD[a], Frederick A. Kuhn, MD, FACS[a,b],*

KEYWORDS

- Sinusitis • Stent • Endoscopic sinus surgery
- Synechiae • Revision endoscopic sinus surgery

The formation of synechiae is the most common complication following endoscopic sinus surgery (ESS). Early series report a rate of 7.5% to 10.5% synechiae formation, with 2.5% to 4% requiring revision surgery.[1,2] Dissection of the frontal recess is the most technically challenging aspect of ESS because of the difficult angle of dissection, the complexity of the frontal recess anatomy, and its relationship to the orbit and cribiform plate. In addition, the frontal sinus is associated with the highest rate of stenosis postoperatively when compared with all other sinuses. Chandra and colleagues[3] reported a 10% stenosis rate when frontal recess dissection was performed. Stents have long been described as an attempt to decrease the rate of synechiae and stenosis.

Stents placed following ESS have five potential functions:

The primary purpose of a stent is to separate edges of a wound surface so as to prevent synechial band formation or stenosis. For example, by not allowing the middle turbinate to make contact with the lateral nasal wall, lateralization of the middle turbinate can be prevented.

Stents also serve to take up space that would otherwise be filled with blood, with fibrin, or with mucus, which would serve as a substrate for unwanted epithelial migration.

In concordance with this, stents can decrease the time and discomfort of postoperative debridement as there is simply less clot/debris to remove.

Stents may also provide a matrix for epithelial migration, especially in areas of denuded bone, as the stent's surface provides subepithelial scar a chance to stabilize.[4]

Finally, stents serve as an occlusive dressing, which has a positive influence on wound healing. Occlusive dressings have been shown to decrease inflammation and necrosis early in wound healing and fibrosis and scarring late in the process.[5]

[a] Georgia Nasal and Sinus Institute, 4750 Waters Avenue, Suite 112, Savannah, GA 31404, USA
[b] Department of Otolaryngology—Head and Neck Surgery, University of North Carolina at Chapel Hill, 101 Manning Drive CB 7070, Chapel Hill, NC 27599-7070, USA
* Corresponding author.
E-mail address: gnsiofficemanager@hotmail.com (F.A. Kuhn).

Otolaryngol Clin N Am 42 (2009) 857–866
doi:10.1016/j.otc.2009.07.001

MIDDLE MEATAL STENTS

As detailed above, the main purposes of stents placed in the middle meatus postoperatively are to decrease synechiae, prevent middle turbinate lateralization, and to fill the ethmoid, which would otherwise be filled with blood, mucus, or fibrin. It is our practice to stent the middle meatus with a "spacer" made from a glove finger, 2-0 silk suture, and a portion of a polyvinyl acetal sponge (Mercocel, Mystic, Connecticut). The sponge is placed inside the glove finger and the two are sutured together and inserted into the middle meatus and inflated with saline.[6] This spacer is smooth and does not adhere to the surrounding tissue, so there is no additional damage to the surrounding tissue upon removal. This technique also prevents the ethmoid from filling with crust and clot, leading to far less postoperative debridement. Finally, the spacer serves as an occlusive dressing that improves wound healing.[7]

Foam made of biodegradable synthetic polyurethane, such as NasoPore (Stryker, Kalamazoo, Michigan), can also be used as a middle meatal stent. This material is initially firm, keeps mucosal surfaces separated, and takes up space in the ethmoid. The material has a hydrophilic component and exposure to water leads to rapid fragmentation of greater than 90% after 5 days.[8] This material can be suitable for patients who cannot tolerate other types of middle meatal stents. However, it is the authors' experience that the material rarely has degraded by 1 week postoperatively. There is also evidence that mucosal healing is initially delayed when compared with a finger-cot stent, but healing appears equal by 3 months postoperatively.[9]

Other middle meatal stents have been described. Shikani[10] detailed a silicone stent with two flanges—one triangular, separating the middle turbinate from the lateral nasal wall, and one smaller, securing the stent in the maxillary sinus. The stent was left in place for 10 to 14 days and results of 50 sides were compared with 50 controls. After a mean follow-up of 8.2 months, patency rate of the stent side was 100% compared with 70% on the control side.[10] This same study design was repeated in a pediatric population, resulting in 10% adhesion formation on the stent side and 55% adhesions on the control side.[11]

FRONTAL SINUS STENTS

The practice of stenting of the frontal sinus has generated debate about several related issues, including type of material, duration, and the basic need for stenting. Outcomes are difficult to evaluate and to compare because of the inherent difficulty of providing for an adequate control. Also, reports have been based on only a few patients, which indicates stenting is generally reserved for a small number of patients.

The first frontal sinus stents were rigid tubes made of various materials. In 1976, Neel and colleagues[12] used a canine model to demonstrate that a thin Silastic (pliable silicone) sheet resulted in less fibrosis, less osteoblastic activity, and more normal mucosal lining when compared with the previously used rigid rubber stents. Numerous prefabricated frontal sinus stents have since been described using silicone. Two examples are the Freeman (InHealth Technologies, Carpinteria, California) and Rains frontal sinus stents (Smith & Nephew ENT, Memphis, Tennessee). The Freeman stent is a biflanged tube and is available in two sizes (14F catheter and 16F catheter). This stent can be inserted via an external incision or endoscopically with an insertion device and a dissolving gel cap for the distal flange. In Freeman's initial report, 6 of 46 patients (13%) failed stenting with restenosis of the frontal sinus after a mean follow-up of 29 months.[13] The Rains frontal sinus stent has a collapsible tapered bulb tip and is available in 4-mm and 6-mm outer diameter sizes. This stent can also be placed endoscopically with a curved suction. In Rains's initial report with a maximum follow-up of

46 months and mean stent duration of 35 days, there was a 94% patency rate.[14] The downside of the prefabricated stents is that they are rigid and cannot adapt to varying ostial diameters (**Fig. 1**). Although reported as flexible, they are much more rigid than traditional Silastic sheeting.

Stents can also be fashioned out of Silastic tubing or sheeting.[15] In our practice, we fabricate stents out of Silastic sheeting varying from 0.01 to 0.04 in thick. The thin sheeting is generally used in three situations:[16]

Tubed in a unilateral frontal sinusotomy when greater than 40% of the mucosa has been denuded
To line a frontal sinus in which a large segment of the mucosa has been disturbed (eg, following tumor removal)
Following a frontal sinus unobliteration

The stents can also be used to aid in frontal recess and ostium debridement. When a Silastic stent is placed in the frontal sinus for 1 week and removed at the first

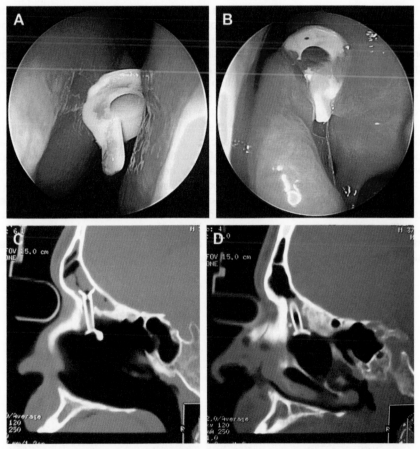

Fig. 1. Example of patient referred to the senior author with prefabricated semirigid silicone stents in place. The patient was referred after stents had been placed and removed four times within the course of 1 year. Endoscopic pictures of stents in place on right (A) and left (B). (C and D) Sagittal CT scans demonstrating stents in place. Note the osteoneogenic bone and the ledge of bone-trapping infection.

debridement, cleaning of the frontal recess and ostium without traumatizing the mucosa is greatly simplified. In these situations, the Silastic conforms to ostium/sinus shape and serves as a matrix or scaffold for mucosal regrowth. **Fig. 2** depicts thin silicone sheeting cut to size for insertion into the frontal sinus. **Fig. 3** demonstrates a 0.01-in thick frontal sinus stent in place 3 months postoperatively and the same frontal sinus 5 months postoperatively in a patient who had severe refractory disease.

The thicker sheeting (0.04 in) can be used to form a U-shaped stent that extends up into the frontal opening as it sits on top of the septum following a Draf III procedure (**Fig. 4**). The Silastic sheeting has numerous advantages as a stenting material. First, it is pliable and easily conforms to the shape of the frontal ostium or frontal sinus. The internal frontal ostium is not a universal shape or size, and therefore a universal stent rarely is a perfect fit. The pliable nature of the material also prevents undue pressure on the sinus mucosa. Finally, the Silastic material may act as an occlusive dressing, which, as previously mentioned, improves tissue healing.

As the duration of stenting increases, more time is allowed for the wound to stabilize and for the mucosal surfaces to remain separated. On the other hand, complications have more potential to occur the longer the stent is left in place (see below). Weber and colleagues,[17] in their excellent review on packing and stents, advocate for a duration of 6 months rather than a particular material. Orlandi and Knight[18] demonstrate that long-term stenting is well tolerated. In their study, nine patients had a mean stenting time of 31.6 months. Orlandi and Knight advocate that stents remain in place until there is an indication for removal (infection or pain). Electron microscopy has demonstrated that, when mucosa is only partially removed, ciliated cells regenerate fully by 6 months following surgery. However, if the mucosa is completely removed, the mucosal regeneration is significantly altered. With complete mucosal disruption, edematous proliferation of granulation occurs, which ultimately results in scar formation. Epithelium then forms after a period of 6 months to 1 year and contains only scattered ciliated cells.[19] Based on this data, one defined stenting period cannot be advocated for all patients. However, if needed, it can be safely done long term. Judgment must be based on the amount of mucosa preserved intraoperatively, and longer stenting times of up to a year are required when there has been complete mucosal disruption.

Now that the types of stents and duration of stenting has been reviewed, the larger question of when to stent, if at all, must be raised. The size of the internal frontal sinus

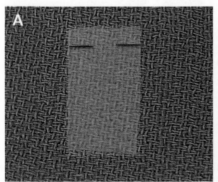
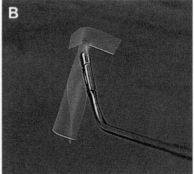

Fig. 2. (*A*) Silastic stent measuring 0.01 in cut into appropriate size. Black line represents location of cuts in the sheet to facilitate stent retention in frontal sinus. (*B*) Same stent rolled and grasped with a 45°giraffe-type forceps for insertion into the frontal sinus.

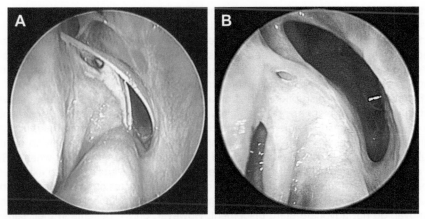

Fig. 3. Left frontal sinus in a patient (*A*) 3 months and (*B*) 5 months postoperatively.

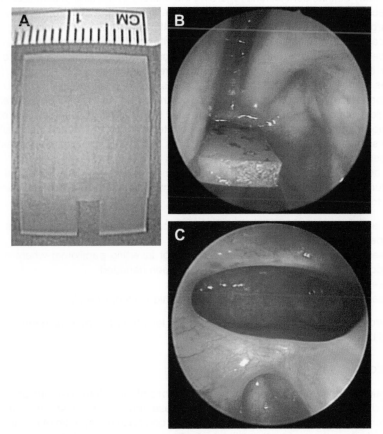

Fig. 4. (*A*) Shape of 0.04-in Silastic stent for Draf III frontal sinusotomy. (*B*) Endoscopic view of right frontal recess with stent in place and seated on septum. (*C*) View of Draf III frontal sinusotomy approximately 4 months following stent removal.

ostium at the completion of the procedure has been the most consistent indication for a stent. Hosemann and colleagues[20] found that a frontal sinusotomy of greater than 5 mm has a stenosis rate of 16% compared with a rate of 33% when the diameter decreases to less than 5 mm. The stenosis rate increases even more to 50% when the diameter is less than 2 mm. Therefore, a frontal ostium size of less than 5 mm should cause the surgeon to pause and consider stent placement.

Extensive mucosal disruption in the frontal sinus or frontal recess is another relative indication for stent placement. When circumferential mucosal disruption is present, most investigators would agree and advocate stent placement to keep the mucosal surfaces apart. The opposite end of the spectrum, however, may not be so clear. Dubin and Kuhn,[16] in their report on frontal sinus osteomas, used a stent when 40% or more of the mucosa was disrupted in the frontal recess. With regards to extended frontal sinus procedures with a drill (Draf IIb or Draf III), there has often been significant mucosal disruption. Kikawada and colleagues,[21] finding restenosis following stent removal, do not advocate stent placement. However, only 4 patients in their series of 22 had a silicone tube stent placed following a Draf IIb or Draf III procedure. One of these 4 patients (25%) had restenosis following stent removal, whereas 5 of 22 patients without stents also had restinosis (22.7%). These numbers are too small to draw any definite conclusions regarding the efficacy of stenting in extended frontal sinus surgery, nor is there a significant difference between the two groups. One study with larger numbers evaluated the use of a Silastic stent for 2 months following a Draf III procedure in 25 patients compared with 39 without. There was no statistical difference between the two groups with regard to frontal ostium patency or symptoms.[22] Weber and colleagues[4] report that stenting prevented stenosis in 15 of 21 (71%) sinuses in their retrospective review using Rains stents, H-shaped silicone tubes, or U-shaped silicone tubes. This study had no control group, so it is difficult to determine if surgical success can be attributed to the stents. This study also represents a complex patient group that has demonstrated refractory disease necessitating aggressive surgical intervention; therefore, a 70% patency can be considered a success.

We advocate stenting with Silastic sheeting in situations where there has been denuded bone or significant disruption of the mucous membrane. This includes any of the following situations:

Cases where greater than 40% of the mucosa in the frontal recess has been denuded

Cases following tumor resection (osteoma or inverting papilloma) where a large portion of the frontal sinus mucosa has been denuded

Cases of frontal sinus unobliteration

Cases involving advanced frontal sinus techniques (eg, Draf III)[23]

In addition, when the frontal sinus ostium is less than 5 mm in diameter, a stent should be considered.

DRUG-CONTAINING STENTS

The enticing concept of combining the benefits of a stent with the benefits of a locally acting drug has been the main focus of stent research over the past few years. This research has explored, for example, the use of corticosteroids, antibiotics, and antineoplastic drugs in combination with stents. Topical corticosteroids have been shown to decrease edema and promote healing following ESS.[7] It is difficult, however, to ensure that topical steroids are able to reach the frontal recess and internal frontal sinus ostium. Therefore, if there were a way to keep mucosal edges separated and apply corticosteroids to decrease edema and expedite wound healing, synechial band formation could be decreased. This also could decrease the need for systemic steroids and the associated complications.

A thin sheet of ethylvinyacetate coated with a film of dexamethasone was successfully used in a group of three patients undergoing an extended frontal sinus procedure. This stent demonstrated that 60 μg of dexamethasone was released per day for 25 days. The stent was well tolerated with no side effects reported and there was only limited follow-up at 3 months.[24] The stent was then evaluated in an animal model, and granulation tissue and stroma thickness were both decreased without affected epithelial differentiation.[25] This system shows promise with the benefits of a Silastic stent combined with the benefits of locally active corticosteroids. Another recent advancement has been the development of a catheter-based system to deploy a microporous reservoir, which gradually moistens the frontal sinus and frontal recess with corticosteroids. The Relieva Stratus Spacer (Acclarent, Menlo Park, California) is placed through a sinus guide into the frontal sinus and 0.32 mL of Kenalog-40 (triamcinolone) is instilled into the reservoir. The device is held in place by nitinol wings and left in place for 2 to 4 weeks postoperatively (**Fig. 5**).

Other medications, besides corticosteroids, have also been investigated. In 2004, Herrmann and colleagues[26] reported on the use of paclitaxel-impregnated stents in sheep. Paclitaxel, an anti-neoplastic compound that stabilizes microtubular arrays and thereby decreases scar formation, was well tolerated in the animal model with no side effects, but no human studies were reported. A group from the Netherlands recently reported on a doxycycline-releasing stent. Doxycycline, a tetracycline antibiotic, was chosen for its antimicrobial effects as well as its ability to affect certain aspects of wound healing, including collagen synthesis and angiogenesis. In this study, the stents were replaced at 1 and 2 months postoperatively and then removed after 3 months and compared with a placebo stent on the opposite side. The doxycycline stents did suppress bacterial growth compared with the placebo stents and endoscopic examination revealed improved healing on the side with the drug-containing stent when evaluated with a visual analog scale.[27] Further research in the realm of drug-containing stents is necessary as there are as of yet no clear-cut results in humans, but these devices show much promise for the future.

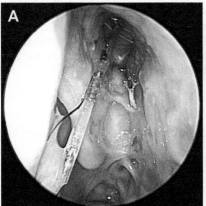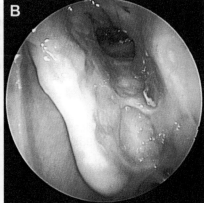

Fig. 5. (A) Left frontal sinus ostium 2 weeks postoperatively with Relieva Stratus Spacer in place. (B) Same frontal sinus immediately following stent removal.

COMPLICATIONS OF NASAL PACKINGS

Toxic shock syndrome (TSS) is a multisystem illness characterized by fever, rash, diarrhea, vomiting, and myalgias. These symptoms can then progress to shock with changes in mental status and hypotension. Initially associated with tampon use in menstruating women, TSS can be associated with any retained foreign body. TSS is caused by TSS toxin I (TSS-1) produced by *Staphylococcus aureus*. Antibiotic prophylaxis has not been shown to be effective in prevention. TSS has been reported in patients with various types of nasal packing as well as in a patient with a Rains frontal sinus stent. Treatment includes removal of the foreign body, a penicillinase-resistant antistaphylococcal antibiotic, and intensive care with hemodynamic support as necessary.[17,28]

Less severe chronic infections are more common in the setting of a sinus stent. Presence of a foreign body in the setting of incompletely healed sinus mucosa (ie, lacking cilia) can predispose these patients to infection. In addition, biofilms readily form on stents with six of six stents demonstrating the presence of a bacterial biofilm in a study by Perloff and Palmer.[29] Culture-directed antibiotics, topical or oral, should be used to control the infection. Chronic infection that is unable to be controlled by medical management may require early stent removal.

It is the authors' experience that when using silicone sheeting as a stenting material, patients need to be followed on a regular basis as a potential complication is migration of the stent into the frontal sinus with resultant stenosis of the ostium. This can then require that the patient return for an additional procedure to remove the stent with a revision frontal sinusotomy. The stent may also migrate out or be blown out by the patient, leading to a shorter duration of stenting than originally desired. To avoid this complication, the stent should be fashioned so that it does not hang into the infundibulum.

SUMMARY: STENTING FOLLOWING ENDOSCOPIC SINUS SURGERY

Stenting following ESS is a complex and somewhat controversial subject. The decision to use or not use a stent is in many cases up to the judgment of the individual surgeon. We are still searching for the ideal stent: one that remains in place; is easily removed, forms an occlusive dressing, but does not exert undue pressure on the mucosa; inhibits bacterial growth as well as scar formation; and decreases edema. There is evidence to suggest, however, that the use of middle meatal finger cot stent improves wound healing, and that frontal sinus stents should be considered when the ostium is less than 5 mm or when there is greater than 40% mucosal disruption in the frontal recess. There has been much innovation with respect to sinus stenting in the past few years, and there is without a doubt more yet to come.

REFERENCES

1. Stankiewicz J. Complications of endoscopic nasal surgery: occurrence and treatment. Am J Rhinol 1987;1:45–9.
2. Gaskins R. Scarring in endoscopic ethmoidectomy. Am J Rhinol 1994;8:271–4.
3. Chandra R, Palmer J, Tangsujarittham T, et al. Factors associated with failure of frontal sinusotomy in the early follow-up period. Otolaryngol Head Neck Surg 2004;131:514–8.
4. Weber R, Mai R, Hosemann W, et al. The success of 6-month stenting in endonasal frontal sinus surgery. Ear Nose Throat J 2000;79:930–41.

5. Alvarez O, Mertz P, Eaglstein W. The effect of occlusive dressings on collagen synthesis and epithelialization in superficial wounds. J Surg Res 1983;35:142–8.
6. Kuhn FA, Citardi MJ. Advances in postoperative care following functional endoscopic sinus surgery. Otolaryngol Clin North Am 1997;30:479–90.
7. Weber R, Keerl R, Huppman A. Investigation of wound healing after paranasal sinus surgery with time lapse video—a pilot study. Am J Rhinol 1996;10: 235–8.
8. Available at: www.polyganics.com/index.php?id=4. Accessed January 5, 2009.
9. Shoman N, Gheriani H, Glamer D, et al. Prospective, double-blind, randomized trial evaluating patient satisfaction, bleeding, and wound healing using biodegradable synthetic polyurethane foam (NasoPore) as a middle meatal spacer in functional endoscopic sinus surgery. J Otolaryngol Head Neck Surg 2009;38: 112–8.
10. Shikani A. A new middle meatal antrostomy stent for functional endoscopic sinus surgery. Laryngoscope 1994;104:638–41.
11. Shikani A. Middle meatal antrostomy stenting following pediatric endoscopic sinus surgery. Am J Rhinol 1996;10:225–8.
12. Neel H, Whitaker J, Lake C. Thin rubber sheeting in frontal sinus surgery: animal and clinical studies. Laryngoscope 1976;86:524–36.
13. Freeman S, Blom E. Frontal sinus stents. Laryngoscope 2000;110(7):1179–82.
14. Rains B. Frontal sinus stenting. Otolaryngol Clin North Am 2001;34(1):101–10.
15. Mirza S, Johnson A. A simple and effective frontal sinus stent. J Laryngol Otol 2000;114:955–6.
16. Dubin M, Kuhn F. Preservation of natural frontal sinus outflow in the management of frontal sinus osteomas. Otolaryngol Head Neck Surg 2006;134:18–24.
17. Weber R, Hochapfel F, Draf W. Packing and stents in endonasal surgery. Rhinology 2000;38:49–62.
18. Orlandi R, Knight J. Prolonged stenting of the frontal sinus. Laryngoscope 2009; 119:190–2.
19. Moriyama H, Yanagi K, Ohtori N, et al. Healing process of sinus mucosa after endoscopic sinus surgery. Am J Rhinol 1996;10:61–6.
20. Hosemann W, Kuhnel T, Held P, et al. Endonasal frontal sinusotomy in surgical management of chronic sinusitis: a critical evaluation. Am J Rhinol 1997;11: 1–19.
21. Kikawada T, Fujigaki M, Kikura M, et al. Extended endoscopic frontal sinus surgery to interrupted nasofrontal communication caused by scarring of the anterior ethmoid: long term results. Arch Otolaryngol Head Neck Surg 1999;125:92–6.
22. Banhiran W, Sargi Z, Collins W, et al. Long term effect of stenting after an endoscopic modified Lothrop procedure. Am J Rhinol 2006;20:595–9.
23. Dubin M, Kuhn F. Endoscopic modified Lothrop (Draf III) with frontal sinus punches. Laryngoscope 2005;115:1702–3.
24. Hosemann W, Schindler E, Wiegrebe E, et al. Innovative frontal sinus stent acting as a local drug-releasing system. Eur Arch Otorhinolaryngol 2003;260:131–4.
25. Beule A, Scharf C, Biebler K, et al. Effects of topically applied dexamethasone on mucosal wound healing using a drug-releasing stent. Laryngoscope 2008;118: 2073–7.
26. Herrmann B, Citardi M, Vogler G, et al. A preliminary report on the effects of Paclitaxel-impregnated stents on sheep nasal mucosa. Am J Rhinol 2004;18:119–24.
27. Huvenne W, Zhang N, Tijsma E, et al. Pilot study using doxycycline-releasing stents to ameliorate postoperative healing quality after sinus surgery. Wound Repair Regen 2008;16:757–67.

28. Chadwell J, Gustafson M, Tami T. Toxic shock syndrome associated with frontal sinus stents. Otolaryngol Head Neck Surg 2001;124:573–4.
29. Perloff J, Palmer J. Evidence of bacterial bioflims on frontal recess stem in patients with chronic rhinosinusitis. Am J Rhinol 2004;18:377–80.

Technical Advances in Rhinologic Basic Science Research

Murugappan Ramanathan, Jr, MD, Justin H. Turner, MD, PhD,
Andrew P. Lane, MD*

KEYWORDS

- Chronic rhinosinusitis • Flow cytometry • Real-time PCR
- Sinonasal epithelial cells • Microarray • Polymorphisms
- Animal models

Chronic rhinosinusitis (CRS) is the single most common self-reported chronic health condition in the United States and is estimated to affect 16% of the adult population annually.[1] Despite the prevalence of this disease, there still exists an incomplete understanding of CRS pathophysiology. Due to the lack of effective therapies directed at CRS refractory to medical and surgical therapy, it is critical that we develop a more mature molecular understanding of CRS and CRS with nasal polyps. Research advances over the years have shifted from CRS emerging from sinus ostial obstruction and persistent bacterial infection to newer mechanisms focusing on inadequate host immune responses, persistent bacterial biofilms, and fungal colonization. Technological advances have helped to embrace many of these new mechanisms. In this review, the authors highlight technological advances in rhinology: real-time polymerase chain reaction, epithelial cell culture, flow cytometry, genomics/single-nucleotide polymorphism detection, microarrays, and genetic/nongenetic animal models of sinusitis. The purpose of this review is to describe these methodologies and their contributions toward achieving a better understanding of CRS.

REAL-TIME PCR

The polymerase chain reaction (PCR) has revolutionized molecular research over the past several decades. PCR is a method that allows exponential amplification of short DNA sequences within a longer double-stranded DNA (dsDNA) and requires the use of primers that are complementary to a defined sequence on each of the 2 strands of DNA. These primers are then extended by a heat stable DNA polymerase (Taq

Division of Rhinology and Sinus Surgery, Department of Otolaryngology-Head and Neck Surgery, The Johns Hopkins School of Medicine, Johns Hopkins Outpatient Center, 6th Floor, 601 N. Caroline Street, Baltimore, MD 21287, USA
* Corresponding author.
E-mail address: alane3@jhmi.edu (A.P. Lane).

Otolaryngol Clin N Am 42 (2009) 867–881
doi:10.1016/j.otc.2009.07.008
0030-6665/09/$ – see front matter © 2009 Published by Elsevier Inc.

oto.theclinics.com

polymerase) to complete the sequence, leading to logarithmic amplification. Historically, PCR products were run on an agarose gel and stained with an ethidium bromide stain because the reaction was qualitative, determining the presence or absence of a product. Another variation of this technique is reverse transcriptase PCR (RT-PCR), which uses the enzyme reverse transcriptase to convert mRNA to cDNA for use in a PCR reaction. Real-time PCR was developed in efforts to quantitatively assess DNA copy number.[2]

Real-Time PCR: the Technique

Real-time PCR has the ability to monitor the progress of PCR as it occurs "in real time." In this technique, reactions are characterized by the point in time during cycling when amplification of a target is first detected, rather than the amount of target accumulated after a fixed number of cycles. The higher the starting copy number of the gene or nucleotide sequence, the sooner a significant increase in fluorescence is detected. In contrast, conventional PCR and RT-PCR measure the amount of accumulated PCR product at the end of the cycle.

Two primary fluorescence-based sequence detection systems are used: Taqman and SYBR Green chemistry. Taqman chemistry uses fluorogenic labeled probes to enable the detection of PCR product as it accumulates. In the Taqman system, specific hybridization between the probe and target is required to generate a fluorescent signal. Probes can also be labeled with different distinguishable reporter dyes, which can allow for amplification of 2 distinct sequences in 1 tube. The primary disadvantage of this system is that specific probes need to be designed for each reaction. SYBR Green dye is a highly specific dye that binds to all dsDNA. As amplicons are created during PCR, SYBR Green binds to all dsDNA causing an increase in fluorescence proportional to the amount of PCR product created (**Fig. 1**). The primary advantage of the SYBR Green system is that no probe is required, which reduces assay time. This system, however, may generate false-positive signals as SYBR Green dye will bind to any dsDNA.

Real-time PCR data are acquired by a computer and can be analyzed in various ways. Cycle thresholds (C_T) reflect the fractional cycle number of a gene or sequence at which the fluorescence passes the fixed threshold, which is a sample that does not contain a template. The ΔC_T method uses the difference in C_T value obtained between a normalizing housekeeping gene (18 S ribosomal RNA, GAPDH) and the target gene to calculate relative quantification (ΔC_T = the difference in threshold cycles for target and housekeeping gene).[3]

Real-Time PCR Applications in Rhinology

Although conventional PCR and RT-PCR have been used for decades in rhinologic research to evaluate for the qualitative presence of markers/genes in nasal tissue, quantitative real-time PCR has largely grown to replace this technique over the past 5 years. Claeys and colleagues[4,5] and Lane and colleagues initially demonstrated the expression of toll-like receptors (TLRs), human beta defensins, and costimulatory molecules from nasal epithelial cells using real-time PCR. Richer and colleagues[6] demonstrated marked reductions in the level of expression of several genes involved in epithelial barrier maintenance and repair in the inflammatory state of CRS. Furthermore, numerous studies have shown altered sinonasal innate immune epithelial gene expression including TLRs, interleukin 22 (IL22), TLRs, and lactoferrin in patients with CRS compared with normal patients.[7–9] Although this literature review is incomplete, it serves to demonstrate that real-time PCR is a powerful rapid method to screen for alterations in genes/markers between control populations and CRS.

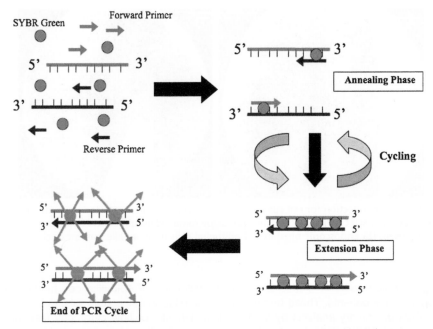

Fig. 1. Real-time PCR using SYBR Green technology. SYBR Green binds to all dsDNA. As primers attach to the denatured strands of DNA, SYBR Green attaches. With continued cycling and extension each newly formed dsDNA will fluoresce, allowing for quantification.

IN VITRO CELL CULTURE SYSTEMS

The hallmark of patient-oriented basic science research is studying the differences between diseased and nondiseased tissue samples. Harvesting sinonasal mucosal biopsies in the operating room is critical to better understanding the cellular and molecular differences in CRS. These tissue biopsies are primarily used either for immunohistochemical staining or to isolate mRNA for PCR. The limitations of these biopsies include small amounts of tissue and the inability to biologically manipulate mucosal cells. Currently, there are no immortalized nasal cell lines from either normal patients or those with CRS. There have been reports of establishing primary nasal fibroblast cultures and of groups using immortalized lower respiratory epithelial cell lines (A549 and BEAS-2B) given the similarities between the upper and lower airways.[10–12]

Primary Sinonasal Epithelial Cells in Culture/Brushed Epithelial Cells

A new advance in rhinologic research has been the use of primary sinonasal epithelial cells (SNECs) grown in culture at the air-liquid interface. This model involves extracting nasal epithelial cells from mucosal biopsies and growing them in cell culture (**Fig. 2**A) as previously described.[5] After these cells reach confluence, they are split into transwell inserts with air above the insert and medium below (**Fig. 3**), mimicking the natural microenvironment of the nose. These cells eventually become ciliated, and histologically resemble fresh brushings of SNECs. Another novel technique to acquire sinonasal tissue is mucosal brush biopsy of the middle meatus, which can be performed in the clinic using topical anesthesia (**Fig. 2**B). The advantage of brushed epithelial cells is that they can be collected easily in the clinic with local anesthesia.

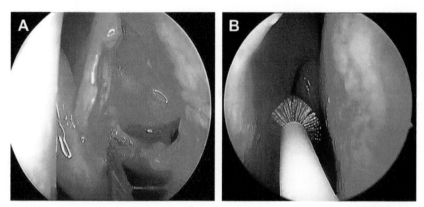

Fig. 2. A tissue collection for cell culture. (*A*) Endoscopic view of a resected uncinate process for isolation of SNECs. Virtually any mucosal tissue removed during endoscopic sinus surgery can be used. (*B*) Endoscopic brushing of epithelial cells in an awake patient in clinic with topical anesthesia.

This technique also facilitates longitudinal evaluation of epithelial cell function in nonoperative patients. These brushings can be used in cell culture or can be used for PCR or primary analysis by immunohistochemistry or flow cytometry (see later discussion). SNECs can be stimulated/suppressed with exogenous cytokines and their effector function can be determined by analyzing the cells for gene/protein expression or the culture medium can be analyzed for secreted proteins.

Recent Advances in Rhinology Research Using SNECs

Numerous investigators have used SNECs from CRS patients in vitro to stimulate the production of cytokines and other effectors. Lalekar and colleagues[13] demonstrated that SNECs can be stimulated with chitin to produce the Th2-associated molecule,

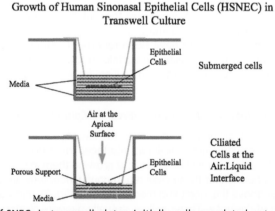

Fig. 3. Growth of SNECs in transwell plates. Initially, cells are plated onto a transwell insert with epithelial growth medium above and below the insert (submerged cells). When these cells reach confluence, the medium above the cells is aspirated. Cells are maintained in this manner until they ciliate, mimicking the natural microenvironment of the nose (air/liquid interface).

acidic mammalian chitinase (AMCase), and eotaxin-3. This finding was the first to suggest the possible existence of an innate immune pathway for local defense against chitin-containing organisms in the sinonasal tract. It is possible that dysregulation of this function could precipitate or exacerbate Th2 inflammation, potentially acting as an underlying factor in CRSwNP. Using SNECs, Kim and colleagues[14] showed that the nasal epithelial costimulatory molecules, B7-H1 and B7-DC, are inducible and elevated in CRS compared with controls. In addition, through using brushed nasal epithelial cells, Saatian and colleagues[15] demonstrated that SNECs express B7-H2 and B7-H3 and may act as antigen-presenting cells to activated mucosal T cells. Clearly, the SNEC model, which mirrors the natural mucosal epithelium of the nose, holds great promise to study the effects of various pharmacologic and environmental stimuli.

FLOW CYTOMETRY

The technique of flow cytometry or fluorescence-activated cell sorting (FACS) has revolutionized single-cell protein analysis and sorting based on cellular protein markers, surface and intracellular. Traditionally, Western blots have been used to measure specific protein expression in cellular or mucosal lysates. The enzyme-linked immunosorbent assay (ELISA) is another technique to measure soluble secreted protein. Unless the tissue source is homogenous, like cell lines, Western blots or ELISA cannot determine which cell type is expressing or secreting a certain protein. Flow cytometry, however, has the powerful ability to sort individual cell populations based on multiple fluorescent markers specific for various receptors or proteins.

Flow Cytometry: the Technique

Flow cytometry uses the principles of light scattering, light excitation, and emission of fluorochrome molecules to generate data from particles and cells. Individual cells and particles are hydrodynamically focused in a sheath of saline before intercepting a focused laser light source. Cell samples are first stained with fluorochrome-conjugated monoclonal antibodies. These stained cells then intercept the light source and scatter light, and fluorochromes are excited to a higher energy state. This energy is then released as a photon of light with specific properties unique to different fluorochromes. Ultimately, flow cytometry measures fluorescence per cell or particle. The analyzed cells can be sorted and collected for further analysis or the data can be stored in the form of a computer file, which can be analyzed as a histogram or quadrant.[16] Most commonly, flow cytometry data are depicted as a 4-quadrant grid with an x and y axis, depicting different fluorochromes (**Fig. 4**). Each cell is depicted as a dot on the plot and its position reflects the fluorochrome intensity. A sample dot plot is shown in **Fig. 4**; 60% of the cells in this brushed cell sample are epithelial cells expressing TLR9.

Recent Rhinologic Advances Using Flow Cytometry

Numerous studies have used flow cytometry to elucidate the pathogenesis of CRS. In 1996, Bernstein and colleagues[17] analyzed different lymphocyte populations in nasal polyps from patients with CRS. This study found that nasal polyp lymphocyte subpopulations may be derived from the local mucosal immune system as well as from random migration of peripheral blood lymphocytes secondary to adhesion molecules and chemokines, which are known to be present in nasal polyps. Conley and colleagues used flow cytometry to measure superantigen-specific T cell receptor domains in the peripheral blood of patients with nasal polyps. This study revealed

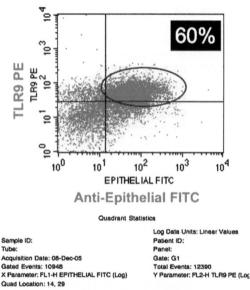

Log Data Units: Linear Values

Sample ID: Patient ID:
Tube: Panel:
Acquisition Date: 08-Dec-05   Gate: G1
Gated Events: 10948   Total Events: 12390
X Parameter: FL1-H EPITHELIAL FITC (Log)   Y Parameter: FL2-H TLR9 PE (Log
Quad Location: 14, 29

Quad	Events	% Gated	% Total	X Mean	X Geo Mean	Y Mean	Y Geo Mean
UL	785	7.17	6.34	7.27	5.90	96.30	52.02
UR	6533	59.67	52.73	83.92	82.27	56.37	51.99
LL	1757	16.05	14.18	6.06	4.93	12.34	9.91
LR	1873	17.11	15.12	67.32	45.59	19.19	17.27

Fig. 4. Example of data acquired through flow cytometry. This sample is a nasal brushing, which contains epithelial cells and other monocytic cells, that was stained for TLR9 PE and antiepithelial cell marker FITC. The upper right corner depicts all cells in this brushing that were positive for both markers (60%).

that 7/12 patients with nasal polyps had a local superantigen effect on T cells.[18] Our group has used flow cytometry extensively to analyze SNECs in control patients and those with CRS with polyps and has shown decreased Toll-like receptor 9 (TLR9) and interleukin 22 receptor (IL22RA-1) levels associated with CRSwNP.[9,19]

MUCOCILIARY CLEARANCE AND CILIARY BEAT FREQUENCY

Ciliary dysfunction is another proposed mechanism for CRS. Respiratory cilia beat in a coordinated manner with a specific frequency and pattern. It is this coordinated beating that clears debris laden mucus toward the natural sinus ostia in a well-established pattern.[20] Studies have shown that stressors such as exercise or infection can alter ciliary beat frequency (CBF). Numerous studies have also shown a decrease in sinonasal mucociliary clearance in CRS patients. Possible reasons for impaired mucus transport include reduced basal CBF and impaired mechanical mucociliary coupling.[21–24]

Measuring CBF

CBF can be measured in vivo using the saccharin transit test or scintigraphy, however these techniques do not take into account regional variations of CBF within the nasal cavity. Also, these studies do not differentiate between the role played by ciliary activity and the overlying mucus blanket. A new advance in measuring CBF has been the advent of high-speed digital microscopy.[25] Numerous groups have developed methods of using digital microscopy and acquisition software. In 2003, Sisson and colleagues[26] developed a fully digital imaging system to quantify CBF accurately and more efficiently compared with analog techniques. Dimova and colleagues[27] adapted a similar system to measure CBF in primary nasal epithelial cells with fast data acquisition and calculation. One area of controversy among in vitro measurements of CBF is the effect of temperature on ciliary function. Some groups take CBF measurements at room temperature, whereas others perform these studies at physiologic body temperature.

To control for the effects of temperature on CBF, Schipor and colleagues[28] developed a novel system using differential interference contrast (DIC) microscopy and to measure CBF at physiologic body temperature. This technique involves placing nasal epithelial cell explants into a temperature-controlled glass perfusion chamber. Microscopic images are visualized using a water immersion objective with DIC optics. Images are then captured using a high-speed monochromatic digital video camera at 250 frames per second. Video images are then analyzed using video imaging processing software on areas of epithelium containing beating cilia, and the frequency is calculated.

Recent Advances Using CBF Measurements

Several investigators have found altered CBF dynamics in CRS patients. Chen and colleagues[29] analyzed CBF in nasal epithelial cells from controls and CRS patients before and after exogenous stimulation with adenosine triphosphate. This study found no differences in basal CBF in controls and CRS patients but found that CRS patients had a minimal increase in CBF after ATP stimulation, concluding that this patient cohort has decreased sinonasal ciliary adaptation to environmental stimuli. Furthermore, Erickson and colleagues[30] used the same method to quantify CBF to demonstrate that retinoic acid is beneficial in ciliary regeneration in stripped maxillary sinus mucosa from rabbits. This study found that CBF was increased in retinoic acid treated mucosa compared with controls. Use of this enhanced technology to measure CBF will allow for a better understanding of how various environmental stimuli affect mucociliary clearance in CRS patients.

SINGLE-NUCLEOTIDE POLYMORPHISM GENOTYPING

It is likely that genetic factors play a role in the pathogenesis of CRS. With the advent of sequencing the human genome, numerous polymorphisms have been associated with chronic disease, including CRS. Polymorphisms are a natural evolutionary process by which multiple phenotypes of a given population are able to exist, resulting in biodiversity and adaptation. Viewed in strictly molecular terms, a polymorphism is an inherited genetic variant that occurs in at least 1% of the human population, excluding spontaneous mutations. Numerous types of polymorphisms exist including single-nucleotide polymorphisms (SNP), restriction fragment length polymorphism (RFLP), and copy number polymorphisms (CNP).[31] An SNP is a DNA sequence variation occurring when a single nucleotide in the genome differs amongst the population. An SNP may occur in the coding region of a gene, thereby altering the amino acid sequence, or it may occur in a noncoding region. Variations in the DNA sequence of a gene can affect susceptibility to disease and how humans respond to pathogens and the environment.

Detecting SNPs: the Technique

Classically, screening for SNPs has employed the use of restriction enzymes, resulting in RFLPs. To examine a population for SNPs, genomic DNA is extracted from either blood or epithelial cells from buccal swabs. Restriction enzymes are bacterial derived enzymes that recognize and cut specific sequences of host or foreign DNA. Most human genes contain dozens of restriction enzyme target sites that, when cleaved, will produce a specific group of DNA fragments of different sizes. This technique allows for single nucleotide changes to be easily detected and for decades has been used as a screening tool to identify disease-associated genetic changes and mutations. With the advent of DNA sequencing, the entire genetic code for a specific protein can now be identified and compared with others in a similar population. New mass spectrometric and DNA microarray technologies also allow for high-throughput analysis of thousands of different single-nucleotide polymorphisms.[32]

Recent Advances: SNPs and CRS

Over the past 3 years, numerous SNPs associated with inflammatory mediators have been examined in CRS patients (**Table 1**). Tewfik and colleagues[33] examined SNPs in the Toll-like receptor 2 (TLR2) gene, which is an innate immune receptor for bacterial lipopolysaccharide, and found no association with an increased incidence in CRS. Similarly, there have also been unsuccessful associations with matrix metalloproteinase 2 and leukotrienes.[34,35] There have been a few positive associations with

Table 1
Single-nucleotide polymorphisms and CRS

Study	Patients	Controls	Findings
Bernstein et al, 2009 (USA)	179 CRSwNP	153 controls	2-fold association with TNF-alpha 308
Castano et al, 2009 (Canada)	206 CRS	196 controls	CRS associated strongly with 5 SNPs of interlekuin-1 receptor-like 1 gene
Endam et al, 2009 (Canada)	206 CRS	196 controls	3 SNPs of interleukin 22 receptor (IL22RA-1) associated with CRS
Cormier et al, 2008 (Canada)	206 CRS	196 controls	No differences in disease with Toll-like receptor 9 (TLR9), but 3 SNPs of TLR9 associated with steroid responsiveness in CRS
De Alarcon et al, 2006 (USA)	51 chronic eosinophilic sinusitis (CHES) 22 ASA 16 chronic inflammatory sinusitis	66 controls	Increased prevalence of A->C base exchange in leukotriene C4 synthase (LTC4S) in CHES
Cheng et al, 2006 (Taiwan)	61 CRSwNP 27 CRS	103 controls	3.39-fold association of CRSwNP and 4.75-fold association of CRS with interlenukin-1 receptor antagonist
Takeuchi et al, 2000 (Japan)	38 CRS	38 controls	74% of CRS patients had tumor necrosis factor B*2 allele

SNPs and CRS progression.[36–42] Bernstein and colleagues examined SNPs in proinflammatory and anti-inflammatory cytokines in control and polypoid CRS patients and found an SNP, TNF-alpha 308, in the promoter region which is associated with a 2-fold increase in developing polypoid CRS. Also, de Alarcon and colleagues found an increased association with leukotriene C4 synthase (LTC4S) and chronic hyperplastic eosinophilic sinusitis. Endam and colleagues found that 3 SNPs of the interleukin 22 receptor (IL22RA-1) have great predisposition to CRS. Although these studies are of low power, they demonstrate a possible genetic basis for certain cases of severe CRS.

DNA MICROARRAYS/GENECHIP

Advances in microtechnology and computer-enhanced laser optics have allowed for the construction of a high-resolution hybridization probe, known as the DNA microarray. The microarray is a carefully constructed set of gene probes to which cDNA copies of RNA expressed within a cell can be hybridized. Computer-enhanced laser detection allows for quantification of this hybridization. The microarray technology uses the knowledge of the sequenced genome and is an extremely comprehensive tool for examining the differential gene expression in various specimens with and without disease.[43]

Microarrays: the Technique

Currently, there are 2 primary methods that are used for microarrays: the GeneChip (Affymetrix Corp) and cDNA microarrays. The Affymetrix GeneChip contains oligo-DNA probes directly synthesized onto glass slides. There are various chips available for different species and subsets of genes, with as many as 47,000 genes. In the cDNA microarray method, cDNA clones are fixed on a glass slide by mechanical microspotting or with noncapillary pens. These arrays can be manufactured in the laboratory and tend to be more expensive and time consuming. In both techniques, RNA samples are allowed to hybridize to the array, and computerized technology detects which probes the target DNA of interest has hybridized with, generating a signal intensity that is quantified.[44] Microarrays are an extremely powerful tool for gene function analysis. Although the functions for most genes on these microarrays are still unknown, some genes still show homology to others with known functions. Although expensive, this technique allows for collection of large amounts of gene expression data with a minimum number of experiments.

Evaluation of Gene Expression in CRS Using Microarrays

Over the past 5 years, 5 major articles have identified causative genes in CRS using gene chip microarrays (**Table 2**). These studies, however, analyzed various disease states within the spectrum of CRS. Anand and colleagues[45] performed the first study in 2006, comparing gene expression using the Affymetrix U133A gene chip in chronic hyperplastic sinusitis and control patients and found 4 specific genes were overexpressed: IL-6, IL-12A, IL-13, and TNF-alpha. However, this study did not differentiate between subclasses of CRS. In 2008, Payne and colleagues[46] performed a small study comparing the unique population of noneosinophilic CRSwNP (n = 2) and controls (n = 2) and found increased expression of IL-6, IL-8, and monocyte chemoattractive protein, and decreased expression of IL-4 and IL-13. Stankovic and colleagues[47] have reported the largest gene chip microarray study thus far, examining 10 patients each with CRSwNP, aspirin sensitive triad asthma polyps, and no disease. This study demonstrated that the CRSwNP phenotype showed

Table 2
Gene chip microarray studies in CRS

Study	Array	Patients/Disease		Genes
Orlandi et al, 2007. Otolaryngol Head Neck Surg	Glass based array 6912 genes	4 allergic fungal sinusitis	3 eosinophilic mucin rhinosinusitis	↑ AFS: cathepsin-B, sialyltransferase 1, GM2 ganglioside protein, S100
Payne et al, 2008. Am J Rhinol	U133 plus 2.0 38,500 genes	2 noneosinophilic CRSwNP	2 controls	↑ IL-6, IL-8, MCP-1, hypoxia induced inflammation, tenascin
Sekigawa et al, 2009. Clin Exp Allergy	Agilent 1a (v2) 17,000 genes	9 aspirin intolerant asthma c NP	5 eisinophilic Rhinosinusitis with NP	↑ IL1R2, INDO
Stankovic et al, 2008. Laryngoscope	U133 plus 2.0 38,500 genes	10 CRSwNP 10 ASA triad	10 controls	↑ c-Met PPPR1 ↓ AZGP1PIP
Anand et al, 2006. Am J Rhinol	U133A 22,000 genes	14 chronic hyperplastic sinusitis	4 control patients	↑ IL-6, IL12-A, IL-13, TNF-alpha

up-regulation of the c-met proto-oncogene and protein phosphatase 1 regulatory subunit and a down-regulation of prolactin-induced protein and zinc alpha2 glyco-protein. Amongst these targets, overexpression of c-Met has been previously impli-cated in nasal polyps.[48] C-Met is a receptor for hepatocyte growth factor, which has been shown to attenuate Th2-associated eosinophilic inflammation. Although there is a great deal of variation in terms of gene expression amongst various investigators, these gene chip microarray studies have uncovered new targets for further investigation.[49,50]

ANIMAL MODELS OF SINONASAL DISEASES

Animal models have allowed scientific investigators to explore human disease processes in ways that could not be safely or ethically performed in human subjects, or that would otherwise be too complex to complete. The increased use of animal models in scientific research comes largely from the perceived limitations of most in vi-tro studies. Many such studies do not replicate the true environment of most biologic reactions and processes. For example, cell culture techniques, particularly those employing transformed cell lines and primary cultures, are typically unable to reproduce complex cell-cell interactions and result in an alteration of the gene expression profile and growth characteristics of their counterparts within live organisms. An animal model is simply defined as any nonhuman animal with a disease or injury that mimics a similar process found in humans. Used extensively for the evaluation, diagnosis, and treatment of a diverse array of pathologic processes, animal models have been a key component in the development of many medications and treatment protocols. Although large animal models (rabbits, dogs, primates) are sometimes used for drug safety and effi-cacy studies, the true workhorse of animal models continues to be the rodent. Mice, in particular, have been used extensively due to their small size and rapid growth rates, as well as the ease by which their genomes can be manipulated.

Nongenetic Animal Models of Sinonasal Diseases

Rodent models of acute and chronic sinonasal diseases have employed several different techniques and have already contributed to our understanding of natural disease course and pathophysiology. Acute rhinosinusitis was first modeled in rabbits 2 decades ago by exposing the maxillary sinus to pathologic bacteria and unilaterally blocking the maxillary sinus ostia.[51] Since that time, the rabbit model of acute sinusitis has been modified and used by multiple investigators. For example, recently Legert and colleagues[52] replicated odontogenic maxillary sinusitis by creating a periapical tooth infection with the rabbit's own oral microflora, followed by histopathological evaluation of sinus mucosa and bone. Two primary mouse models of acute rhinosinusitis have been reported in the literature. Bomer and colleagues[53] developed a model of acute rhinosinusitis by intranasally inoculating mice with *Streptococcus pneumoniae*. This particular model has since been used by multiple groups and has even been modified to more closely resemble acute fungal rhinosinusitis and chronic rhinosinusitis.[54] A model for acute viral rhinosinusitis was reported by Klemens and colleagues[55] In this example, mice were nasally inoculated with Sendai virus resulting in an acute viral infection that resolved spontaneously within 10 days.

The complexity inherent in modeling a chronic disease process has resulted in fewer successful models of chronic sinonasal disease. As with the acute disease, the first models of CRS were developed in rabbits. Kumlien and Schiratzki[56] induced chronic sinonasal inflammation by nasal inoculation with *Streptococcus pneumonia* and placement of a foreign body in the maxillary sinus. This model has since been used and modified several times, with most recent models being developed instead in mice. Jacob and colleagues[57] were able to induce a persistent, localized bacterial sinusitis in mice either by unilateral maxillary sinus ostium obstruction with merocel nasal packing, or by inoculation with *Bacillus fragilis*. The use of *Steptococcus pneumonia* inoculation to model allergic CRS was later modified by Wang and colleagues,[58] who combined bacterial inoculation with unilateral ostiomeatal obstruction with merocel to more accurately model the chronic disease.

The development of a murine model of chronic eosinophilic rhinosinusitis was reported by Bolger's group in 2006.[59] These mice were sensitized to *Aspergillus fumigates* extract via intraperitoneal injection and then by repeated nasal challenges, resulting in the creation of a consistent inflammatory response. A similar allergic CRS model was reported by Hussain and colleagues[60] These mice were sensitized with intraperitoneal injection with ovalbumin followed by repeated intranasal ovalbumin injection over a 12-week period. The bacterial CRS murine systems have thus far been able to successfully model the distinct immunologic characteristics of these closely related diseases. Research into atopic diseases such as asthma and allergic rhinitis has also been aided by mouse models. Classic models have been produced by intraperitoneal injection of a sensitizing agent into mice, which results in the rapid proliferation of Th2 helper T cells and allergen-specific IgE. The atopic response can then be modeled by nebulizer or intranasal exposure to allergen.

GENETIC ANIMAL MODELS OF SINONASAL DISEASES: TRANSGENIC/KNOCK-OUT MICE

The first transgenic mouse was created in 1982.[61] Since that time, transgenic mice have become priceless models for studying human diseases and their treatments. A transgenic organism has had a foreign gene deliberately inserted into its genome. The production of a transgenic organism begins with the isolation of a specific gene. There are then 2 methods by which a transgenic organism can be created. In the first, the gene of interest is injected into fertilized embryos, which are subsequently implanted into a pseudopregnant female. A certain percentage of the offspring will be expected to express the gene of interest as heterozygotes. Two heterozygotes can then be mated, which will result in approximately 1 out of 4 offspring being homozygous for the gene of interest. In the second method, embryonic stem cells harvested from the inner cell mass of blastocysts are grown in culture and transformed with the gene of interest. Successfully transformed cells are then reimplanted into a blastocyst and introduced into a pseudopregnant female. Selecting for homozygotes is then performed in the same fashion. Genes can be inserted either randomly or targeted to a particular region in the genome. Endogenous genes can be replaced with nonfunctioning gene sequences to produce a "knock-out" mouse. In some situations "knock-in" or "knock-out" of a certain gene is only desired in specific tissues or cell types. Systems now exist by which "target" genes can be activated only in specific cells, and in a temporally controlled manner. Although mice have been the most commonly used transgenic animals, transgenics have now also been created in pigs, sheep, chickens, and most recently primates.

The use of transgenic and genetically modified animals in rhinologic research has thus far been limited. In a hybrid experiment investigating the adoptive transfer hypothesis, Kanaizumi and colleagues[62] generated Th0, Th1, and Th2 cells in DO11.10 transgenic mice, which express an ovalbumin(OVA)-specific T cell receptor. These immunoresponsive T cells were then transferred into wild-type BALB/c mice. Following nasal OVA challenge only Th2 cells were recruited to the nasal mucosa, supporting an important role for Th2 responses in allergic rhinitis. Recently, Lane and colleagues[63] have developed a transgenic mouse model for human chronic rhinosinusitis-associated olfactory dysfunction. Termed the inducible olfactory inflammation (IOI) mouse, this model uses a doxycycline-inducible tet-regulated activation system to permit spatially and temporally controlled expression of any target gene. By expressing TNF-α within mouse olfactory epithelium they were able to produce histopathologic evidence of local inflammation that could be maintained for a period of months, and which resulted in loss of olfactory function. Many different transgenic animals have been created with the purpose of exploring individual components of immunologic pathways involved in asthma, allergy, and inflammation. Although used sparingly thus far in rhinologic research, the use of transgenic animals may ultimately augment our understanding of a multitude of sinonasal diseases.

THE FUTURE OF RHINOLOGIC BASIC SCIENCE RESEARCH

Over the past decade, molecular and cellular technical advances have helped to achieve a better understanding of CRS. In the next decade, it is anticipated that more definitive animal models of CRS will be available to further characterize the pathogenesis of the disease state. Also, a more mature understanding of the epigenetic modifications that sustain Th2 dysregulation in CRSwNP will be necessary. In conclusion, scientific advancements in molecular and genomic technology will continue to benefit the rhinologist investigator in achieving a better understanding of CRS, ultimately leading to more effective pharmacologic interventions in the future.

REFERENCES

1. Anand VK. Epidemiology and economic impact of chronic rhinosinusitis. Ann Otol Rhinol Laryngol Suppl 2004;193:3–5.

2. Williams PM. The beginnings of real-time PCR. Clin Chem 2009;55(4):833–4.
3. Essentials of real-time PCR. Product insert. Applied Biosystems; 2006.
4. Claeys S, de Belder T, Holtappels G, et al. Human beta-defensins and toll-like receptors in the upper airway. Allergy 2003;58(8):748–53.
5. Lane AP, Saatian B, Yu XY, et al. mRNA for genes associated with antigen presentation are expressed by human middle meatal epithelial cells in culture. Laryngoscope 2004;114(10):1827–32.
6. Richer SL, Truong-Tran AQ, Conley DB, et al. Epithelial genes in chronic rhinosinusitis with and without nasal polyps. Am J Rhinol 2008;22(3):228–34.
7. Lane AP, Truong-Tran QA, Myers A, et al. Serum amyloid A, properdin, complement 3, and toll-like receptors are expressed locally in human sinonasal tissue. Am J Rhinol 2006;20(1):117–23.
8. Psaltis AJ, Bruhn MA, Ooi EH, et al. Nasal mucosa expression of lactoferrin in patients with chronic rhinosinusitis. Laryngoscope 2007;117(11):2030–5.
9. Ramanathan M Jr, Spannhake EW, Lane AP. Chronic rhinosinusitis with nasal polyps is associated with decreased expression of mucosal interleukin 22 receptor. Laryngoscope 2007;117(10):1839–43.
10. Nonaka M, Pawankar R, Fukumoto A, et al. Induction of eotaxin production by interleukin-4, interleukin-13 and lipopolysaccharide by nasal fibroblasts. Clin Exp Allergy 2004;34(5):804–11.
11. Wang JH, Kwon HJ, Lee BJ, et al. Staphylococcal enterotoxins A and B enhance rhinovirus replication in A549 cells. Am J Rhinol 2007;21(6):670–4.
12. Heinecke L, Proud D, Sanders S, et al. Induction of B7-H1 and B7-DC expression on airway epithelial cells by the toll-like receptor 3 agonist double-stranded RNA and human rhinovirus infection: in vivo and in vitro studies. J Allergy Clin Immunol 2008;121(5):1155–60.
13. Lalaker A, Nkrumah L, Lee WK, et al. Chitin stimulates expression of acidic mammalian chitinase and eotaxin-3 by human sinonasal epithelial cells in vitro. Am J Rhinol Allergy 2009;23(1):8–14.
14. Kim J, Myers AC, Chen L, et al. Constitutive and inducible expression of b7 family of ligands by human airway epithelial cells. Am J Respir Cell Mol Biol 2005;33(3):280–9. Epub 2005 Jun 16.
15. Saatian B, Yu XY, Lane AP, et al. Expression of genes for B7-H3 and other T cell ligands by nasal epithelial cells during differentiation and activation. Am J Physiol Lung Cell Mol Physiol 2004;287(1):L217–25.
16. Brown M, Wittwer C. Flow cytometry: principles and clinical applications in hematology. Clin Chem 2000;46(8 Pt 2):1221–9.
17. Bernstein JM, Ballow M, Rich G, et al. Lymphocyte subpopulations and cytokines in nasal polyps: is there a local immune system in the nasal polyp? Otolaryngol Head Neck Surg 2004;130(5):526–35.
18. Conley DB, Tripathi A, Seiberling KA, et al. Superantigens and chronic rhinosinusitis: skewing of T-cell receptor V beta-distributions in polyp-derived CD4+ and CD8+ T cells. Am J Rhinol 2006;20(5):534–9.
19. Ramanathan M Jr, Lee WK, Dubin MG, et al. Sinonasal epithelial cell expression of toll-like receptor 9 is decreased in chronic rhinosinusitis with polyps. Am J Rhinol 2007;21(1):110–6.
20. Messerklinger W. Direction of ciliary flow on the mucosa of the upper respiratory tract. Z Laryngol Rhinol Otol 1951;30:302–8.
21. Sanderson MJ, Dirksen ER. Mechanosensitivity of cultured ciliated cells from the mammalian respiratory tract: implications for the regulation of mucociliary transport. Proc Natl Acad Sci U S A 1986;83:7302–6.

22. Sanderson MJ, Dirksen ER. Mechanosensitive and beta-adrenergic control of the ciliary beat frequency of mammalian respiratory tract cells in culture. Am Rev Respir Dis 1989;139:432–40.

23. Mwimbi XK, Muimo R, Green MW, et al. Making human nasal cilia beat in the cold: a real time assay for cell signalling. Cell Signal 2003;15:395–402.

24. Majima Y, Sakakura Y, Matsubara T, et al. Possible mechanisms of reduction of nasal mucociliary clearance in chronic sinusitis. Clin Otolaryngol 1986;11: 55–60.

25. Sanderson MJ. High-speed digital microscopy. Methods 2000;21:325–34.

26. Sisson JH, Stoner JA, Ammons BA, et al. All-digital image capture and whole-field analysis of ciliary beat frequency. J Microsc 2003;211(Pt 2):103–11.

27. Dimova S, Maes F, Brewster ME, et al. High-speed digital imaging method for ciliary beat frequency measurement. J Pharm Pharmacol 2005;57(4):521–6.

28. Schipor I, Palmer JN, Cohen AS, et al. Quantification of ciliary beat frequency in sinonasal epithelial cells using differential interference contrast microscopy and high-speed digital video imaging. Am J Rhinol 2006;20(1):124–7.

29. Chen B, Shaari J, Claire SE, et al. Altered sinonasal ciliary dynamics in chronic rhinosinusitis. Am J Rhinol 2006;20(3):325–9.

30. Erickson VR, Antunes M, Chen B, et al. The effects of retinoic acid on ciliary function of regenerated sinus mucosa. Am J Rhinol 2008;22(3):334–6.

31. Mein CA, Barratt BJ, Dunn MG, et al. Evaluation of single nucleotide polymorphism typing with invader on PCR amplicons and its automation. Genome Res 2000;10(3):330–43.

32. Ohnishi Y, Tanaka T, Ozaki K, et al. A high-throughput SNP typing system for genome-wide association studies. J Hum Genet 2001;46(8):471–7.

33. Tewfik MA, Bossé Y, Hudson TJ, et al. Assessment of toll-like receptor 2 gene polymorphisms in severe chronic rhinosinusitis. J Otolaryngol Head Neck Surg 2008;37(4):552–8.

34. Wang LF, Chien CY, Kuo WR, et al. Matrix metalloproteinase-2 gene polymorphisms in nasal polyps. Arch Otolaryngol Head Neck Surg 2008;134(8):852–6.

35. Al-Shemari H, Bossé Y, Hudson TJ, et al. Influence of leukotriene gene polymorphisms on chronic rhinosinusitis. BMC Med Genet 2008;9:21.

36. Bernstein JM, Anon JB, Rontal M, et al. Genetic polymorphisms in chronic hyperplastic sinusitis with nasal polyposis. Laryngoscope 2009;119(7):1258–64.

37. de Alarcón A, Steinke JW, Caughey R, et al. Expression of leukotriene C4 synthase and plasminogen activator inhibitor 1 gene promoter polymorphisms in sinusitis. Am J Rhinol 2006;20(5):545–9.

38. Cheng YK, Lin CD, Chang WC, et al. Increased prevalence of interleukin-1 receptor antagonist gene polymorphism in patients with chronic rhinosinusitis. Arch Otolaryngol Head Neck Surg 2006;132(3):285–90.

39. Takeuchi K, Majima Y, Sakakura Y. Tumor necrosis factor gene polymorphism in chronic sinusitis. Laryngoscope 2000;110(10 Pt 1):1711–4.

40. Castano R, Bosse Y, Endam LM, et al. Evidence of association of interleukin-1 receptor-like 1 gene polymorphisms with chronic rhinosinusitis. Am J Rhinol Allergy 2009;23(4):377–84.

41. Cormier C, Bosse Y, Tewfik M, et al. Polymorphisms in TLR9 gene influence response to corticosteroids in severe chronic rhinosinusitis [abstract]. J Allergy Clin Immunol 2008;121(2 Suppl 1):S218.

42. Endam L, Bossé Y, Filali-Mouhim A. Polymorphisms in the interleukin-22 receptor alpha-1 gene are associated with severe chronic rhinosinusitis [abstract]. AAO Meeting. Chicago (IL), September 16–19, 2008.

43. Li X, Quigg RJ, Zhou J, et al. Clinical utility of microarrays: current status, existing challenges and future outlook. Curr Genomics 2008;9(7):466–74.
44. Dufva M. Introduction to microarray technology. Methods Mol Biol 2009;529:1–22.
45. Anand VK, Kacker A, Orjuela AF, et al. Inflammatory pathway gene expression in chronic rhinosinusitis. Am J Rhinol 2006;20(4):471–6.
46. Payne SC, Han JK, Huyett P, et al. Microarray analysis of distinct gene transcription profiles in non-eosinophilic chronic sinusitis with nasal polyps. Am J Rhinol 2008;22(6):568–81.
47. Stankovic KM, Goldsztein H, Reh DD, et al. Gene expression profiling of nasal polyps associated with chronic sinusitis and aspirin-sensitive asthma. Laryngoscope 2008;118(5):881–9.
48. Rho HS, Lee SH, Lee HM, et al. Overexpression of hepatocyte growth factor and its receptor c-Met in nasal polyps. Arch Otolaryngol Head Neck Surg 2006; 132(9):985–9.
49. Orlandi RR, Thibeault SL, Ferguson BJ. Microarray analysis of allergic fungal sinusitis and eosinophilic mucin rhinosinusitis. Otolaryngol Head Neck Surg 2007;136(5):707–13.
50. Sekigawa T, Tajima A, Hasegawa T, et al. Gene-expression profiles in human nasal polyp tissues and identification of genetic susceptibility in aspirin-intolerant asthma. Clin Exp Allergy 2009;39(7):972–81.
51. Drettner B, Johansson P, Kumlien J. Experimental acute sinusitis in rabbit. A study of mucosal blood flow. Acta Otolaryngol 1987;103(5–6):432–4.
52. Legert KG, Melén I, Heimdahl A, et al. Development and characterization of an animal model of dental sinusitis. Acta Otolaryngol 2005;125(11):1195–202.
53. Bomer K, Brichta A, Baroody F, et al. A mouse model of acute bacterial sinusitis. Arch Otolaryngol Head Neck Surg 1998;124(11):1227–32.
54. Rodriguez TE, Falkowski NR, Harkema JR, et al. Role of neutrophils in preventing and resolving acute fungal sinusitis. Infect Immun 2007;75(12):5663–8.
55. Klemens JJ, Thompson K, Langerman A, et al. Persistent inflammation and hyperresponsiveness following viral rhinosinusitis. Laryngoscope 2006;116(7):1236–40.
56. Kumblien J, Schiratzki H. Blood flow in the rabbit sinus mucosa during experimentally induced chronic sinusitis. Measurement with a diffusible and with a non-diffusible tracer. Acta Otolaryngol 1985;99(5–6):630–6.
57. Jacob A, Faddis BT, Chole RA. Chronic bacterial rhinosinusitis: description of a mouse model. Arch Otolaryngol Head Neck Surg 2001;127(6):657–64.
58. Wang H, Lu X, Cao PP, et al. Histological and immunological observations of bacterial and allergic chronic rhinosinusitis in the mouse. Am J Rhinol 2008;22(4):343–8.
59. Lindsay R, Slaughter T, Britton-Webb J, et al. Development of a murine model of chronic rhinosinusitis. Otolaryngol Head Neck Surg 2006;134(5):724–30.
60. Hussain I, Randolph D, Brody SL, et al. Induction, distribution and modulation of upper airway allergic inflammation in mice. Clin Exp Allergy 2001;31(7):1048–59.
61. Palmiter RD, Brinster RL, Hammer RE, et al. Dramatic growth of mice that develop from eggs microinjected with metallothionein-growth hormone fusion genes. Nature 1982;300(5893):611–5.
62. Kanaizumi E, Shirasaki H, Sato J, et al. Establishment of animal model of antigen-specific T lymphocyte recruitment into nasal mucosa. Scand J Immunol 2002; 56(4):376–82.
63. Lane AP, Turner JH, May L. Reversible loss of neuronal marker protein expression in a transgenic mouse model for sinusitis-associated olfactory dysfunction [abstract]. American Rhinologic Society Meeting-COSM. Orlando (FL), May 1–2, 2008.

Technologic Innovations in Neuroendoscopic Surgery

Carl H. Snyderman, MD[a,b,*], Ricardo L. Carrau, MD[a,b],
Daniel M. Prevedello, MD[b], Paul Gardner, MD[b],
Amin B. Kassam, MD[c]

KEYWORDS

• Skull base surgery • Neuroendoscopy • Technology • Imaging

Technology often drives progress, and that is true with endoscopic surgery of the cranial base. The introduction of endoscopes and endoscopic instruments for the treatment of sinus disease paved the way for more advanced surgeries that extended the limits of surgery to the orbit, ventral skull base, and upper cervical spine. There are unique technologic challenges with the endoscopic endonasal skull base surgery, such as a limited working space, difficulty in visualization and identification of neurovascular structures and removal of tissue, hemostasis, and dural reconstruction. Some of the technologic challenges of endonasal skull base surgery were met through simple modifications of existing sinus surgery instruments. Others are still limiting factors for continued progress. Technologic advances that have enabled this surgery include specialized operating suites, neurophysiologic monitoring, imaging and visualization technologies, powered instrumentation, hemostatic materials, and reconstructive materials.

OPERATING SUITE

A specialized operating suite offers multiple enhancements for the benefit of the patient, surgeons, anesthesiologist, and other medical personnel. Access to the patient is facilitated by suspending equipment from booms mounted onto the ceiling.

[a] Department of Otolaryngology-Head and Neck Surgery, University of Pittsburgh School of Medicine, 200 Lothrop St, Pittsburgh, PA 15213, USA.
[b] Department of Neurosurgery, University of Pittsburgh School of Medicine, 200 Lothrop St, Pittsburgh, PA 15213, USA.
[c] St John's Health Center, John Wayne Cancer Institute, 2200 Santa Monica Blvd, Santa Monica, CA 90404, USA
* Corresponding author. Department of Otolaryngology-Head and Neck Surgery, University of Pittsburgh School of Medicine, 200 Lothrop St, Pittsburgh, PA 15213, USA.
E-mail address: snydermanch@upmc.edu (C.H. Snyderman).

Otolaryngol Clin N Am 42 (2009) 883–890
doi:10.1016/j.otc.2009.08.019
oto.theclinics.com

Multiple monitors provide both surgeons with comfortable viewing angles (**Fig. 1**). Wall-mounted screens allow the operative assistants and anesthesiologists to monitor the progress of the surgery and respond appropriately to a surgical crisis. A telestration monitor facilitates communication between the surgeons and observing physicians who are learning. Anatomic structures can be highlighted, and directions provided. Other data are also imported into the screens to allow the surgeon to track multiple physiologic processes simultaneously, such as vital signs, neurophysiologic monitoring, and radiologic imaging.

NEUROPHYSIOLOGIC MONITORING

Neurophysiologic monitoring provides complete monitoring of the intraoperative environment.[1] Modalities include somatosensory evoked potentials (SSEPs), brainstem evoked responses (BSERs), cranial nerve electromyography, and microvascular Doppler. SSEP consists of simultaneous stimulation of upper (median) and lower (tibial) extremity peripheral nerves, with monitoring of cortical brain responses. SSEP is a sensitive method of assessing the adequacy of hemispheric blood flow during carotid manipulation or injury. It also provides information concerning brainstem function and integrity. Inadequate perfusion (hypotension), especially during blood loss, can be detected by SSEP in the absence of other physiologic changes. SSEPs are monitored in all skull base surgeries because of the potential for carotid injury and major venous bleeding from the cavernous sinus. In rare cases, SSEP

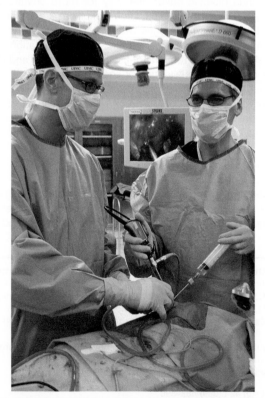

Fig. 1. An operating suite dedicated to neuroendoscopy integrates different types of visual data and makes them accessible to the entire operating team.

monitoring can alert the surgeon to developing complications, such as intracranial hemorrhage, and allow early intervention before a clinical examination or imaging.

BSER provides similar monitoring of brainstem function and is used during surgery in the region of the brainstem (transclival approach), especially when there is tumor compression of the brainstem. Electromyography of the cranial nerves provides information regarding the integrity of the cranial nerves and can detect manipulation of the nerve before injury. Stimulation of tumor tissues with an endoscopic probe during dissection can help localize the nerve and avoid injury. A microvascular Doppler is used to identify vessels such as the internal carotid artery (ICA) when it is displaced from its normal location or obscured by a tumor or scar tissue.

IMAGING

Image guidance or intraoperative navigation is an essential technology for endonasal skull base surgery. The skull base is a "black box" and the location of important neurovascular structures is not always readily apparent. Preoperative computed tomography (CT) angiography provides good definition of bone structures and the ICA. Magnetic resonance imaging (MRI) provides better soft tissue detail, especially when there is intracranial extension. If both types of information are needed, image fusion is performed. Image guidance is used to identify normal anatomic structures, detect tumor margins, and assess the completeness of resection.

One drawback of image guidance technology is the absence of real-time imaging. Static images reflect the preoperative status of the patient. With large intracranial tumors, shift of soft tissues after debulking of the tumor renders the image guidance information regarding the tumor-brain interface inaccurate. The images can be updated with an intraoperative CT or MRI scanner with minimal delay (**Fig. 2**). This allows the surgeon to assess the completeness of resection, detect movement of structures, and complete the tumor resection if warranted. In rare cases, an intraoperative scan can detect complications such as intracranial hemorrhage (eg, subdural hematoma) and allow surgical intervention before the patient leaves the operating room.

VISUALIZATION

There are no dramatic changes in endoscopic visualization since the introduction of the rod lens endoscope. Several angled endoscopes are available to increase the field

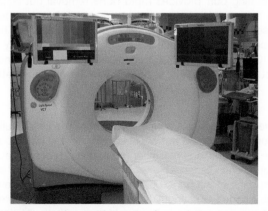

Fig. 2. Intraoperative CT provides rapid imaging for updating image guidance, assessment of tumor resection, and early detection of complications.

of vision. A wide-angle endoscope may provide even greater field of view with minimal distortion. The quality of visual display has been enhanced with the introduction of high-definition cameras and plasma screens.

One perceived deficiency of endoscopic visualization is the lack of 3-dimensional (3D) imaging. In reality, the human brain adapts quickly to a 2D environment and there are abundant visual cues during endoscopic surgery that contribute to a pseudo-3D perception. Past efforts to create a 3D endoscope were limited by the size constraints of the endoscope and the physical need to separate 2 viewing channels as much as possible. Innovative technology now allows the placement of a 3D chip on the tip of the endoscope, thus rendering true 3D views.[2] Whether such views offer any real advantage for the surgeon remains to be seen.

The greatest area for development with visualization is the visual display of information. The surgeon is bombarded with different types of information in the surgical environment. Visual displays can be merged to provide the surgeon with 1 display containing the endoscopic view, preoperative scans, image guidance, vital signs, and neurophysiologic monitoring. Future developments will present this in a heads up display that is interactive and customizable for the surgeon.

DISSECTION

Dissecting instruments are predominantly modifications of standard surgical instruments. Increased lengths and angles and a smaller diameter make them suitable for intranasal use. Tools for soft tissue dissection include malleable suctions, blunt dissectors, angled rotatable scissors, and through-cutting instruments. Although microdebriders are suitable for tumor debulking, they are considered too aggressive for dissection close to nerves and vessels. Ultrasonic aspirators modified for endonasal surgery can be used to debulk tumors, but they generate excessive heat and can cause thermal injury to the nasal tissues and adjacent neural and vascular structures. Fiberoptic and wave-guided lasers were used successfully to incise soft tissues but were again limited by potential heat generation or tissue necrosis in proximity to a vessel or nerve and injury to deep structures.

Removal of the bone of the cranial base is one of the more challenging aspects of cranial base surgery because of the amount of bone removal that is sometimes necessary and the proximity to important neural and vascular structures. Endonasal drills are available with straight and angulated tips and can be incorporated into the navigational system. A cutting burr provides rapid bone removal but lacks precision and does not provide hemostasis. A diamond burr is good for bone hemostasis but is too tedious to use and generates a lot of heat. A combination hybrid or coarse diamond bit contains the best features of both burrs and allows very precise removal of bone over the ICA or optic nerve. Ultrasonic aspirators with bone-dissecting tips remove bone through rapid oscillations of the tip and are an alternative to drills.[3]

HEMOSTASIS

Hemostasis is one of the biggest concerns during endonasal skull base surgery.[4] Monopolar electrocautery should not be used beyond the nasal cavity because of the risk of injury to neural and vascular structures. Bipolar electrocautery with a pistol-grip design is an indispensable tool for the cauterization of soft tissue, small vessels, and the surface of the dura. Endoscopic bipolars have interchangeable tips with different sizes, shapes, and angulations to accommodate different clinical situations (Fig. 3). Venous hemostasis is best achieved with the topical application of various hemostatic materials, such as gelatin sponge, oxidized regenerated cellulose,

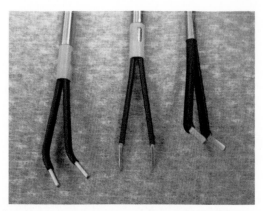

Fig. 3. Endoscopic bipolar electrocautery is an indispensable tool for precise hemostasis and is available with interchangeable tips for different clinical situations.

microfibrillar collagen, topical thrombin, and fibrin sealant. These are effective for bleeding from the cavernous sinus but need to be applied properly. Syvek (Marine Polymer Technologies, Inc, Danvers, MA, USA) is a hemostatic patch derived from plankton, which promotes platelet aggregation and clotting and is applied to a bleeding arterial wall for several minutes and then removed.[5] It may be effective for small puncture wounds or arterioles. Every endoscopic surgeon should be aware of the hemostatic effects of warm saline irrigation. Stangerup and colleagues[6] showed that hot water irrigation is an effective treatment for the management of epistaxis. The authors use a hot water bath intraoperatively to maintain saline at 40°C. Irrigation of the nasal cavity is effective for diffuse mucosal oozing and minor bleeding from the surface of the tumor or brain and can avoid unnecessary application of hemostatic material to fragile tissues. Other hemostatic materials are being developed but do not appear to offer any significant advantages over the methods described here.

Injury to the ICA can be catastrophic if not handled properly. A small hole from the avulsion of an arteriole can be sealed using bipolar electrocautery or by application of hemostatic material, such as oxycellulose and fibrin glue. A larger laceration requires sacrifice of the vessel. Intraoperatively, this can be accomplished with focal packing or the application of aneurysm clips. Postoperatively, the injury can be treated with endovascular techniques with preservation (vascular stenting) or sacrifice (coiling) of the vessel.

RECONSTRUCTION

Reconstruction of large dural defects is one of the greatest challenges of endonasal skull base surgery.[7] Standard techniques using inlay and onlay fascial grafts resulted in an unacceptable rate of postoperative cerebrospinal fluid (CSF) leaks. Several technologic innovations have reduced the overall CSF leak rate to less than 5%.[8] Various dural substitutes are now available. These dural substitutes are thin and pliable, but absorbable products can be porous. They can be used as a single layer for dural reconstruction over the convexity of the cranium but will leak if used endonasally. They make a good inlay graft when used endonasally but require covering with a nonporous material or mucosal flap. Alternatives to autologous fascial grafts include cadaveric dura or pericardium and processed cadaveric dermis. Although direct suturing of fascial grafts to achieve a watertight seal has been described, it is

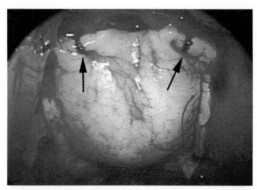

Fig. 4. A nitinol U-clip (Medtronic) facilitates direct suturing of fascial grafts.

technically difficult. Instead, several sutures can be placed to hold a graft in place so that it is not displaced by a fat graft or flap. This technical exercise is greatly simplified with the use of the Medtronic U-clip (Medtronic, Minneapolis, MN, USA), a vascular suture made from nitinol (metal with memory).[9] After the needle is passed, the nitinol segment is detached and it coils on itself to hold the graft securely (**Fig. 4**). The greatest advance in dural reconstruction is the adaptation of the septal mucosal flap as described by Hadad and colleagues.[10] This vascularized flap is large enough to reconstruct defects extending from orbit to orbit and from the frontal sinus to the sella (**Fig. 5**). Tissue glues can be used to hold materials in place or provide a protective barrier. Although fibrin glue can be created from the patient's own serum, commercially prepared fibrin glues made from pooled serum are far superior. In the absence of a CSF leak, fibrin glue provides some hemostasis and a protective covering for exposed dura or pituitary gland while the tissues heal. Growth factors in the fibrin glue may actually hasten the healing process. Synthetic glues provide a more long-lasting barrier and are used to cover the dural reconstruction. Rigid materials

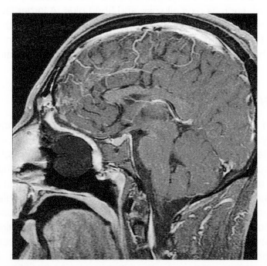

Fig. 5. MRI of septal flap shows coverage from the frontal sinus to the sella.

can be used as part of the reconstruction to hold fascial or fat grafts in place. These include titanium plates and absorbable mesh. The authors do not recommend their use because of the risks of migration and vascular injury and infection. Similarly, hydroxyapatite bone cement is not used for reconstruction because of the risk of infection.

FUTURE TECHNOLOGIES

There will continue to be minor refinements in surgical tools and existing technologies. New materials for hemostasis and dural reconstruction will be introduced. Some of the future needs are already described. The next major revolution in surgical technology will probably be in robotics. New robotic technologies will enable simultaneous surgery by multiple surgeons, provide greater access to hard-to-reach areas, and enhance manual dexterity. Multiport surgery using multiple simultaneous corridors will provide optimal access with minimal displacement of normal neural and vascular structures. The introduction of robotic technology will be accompanied by the increased use of simulation for visualization of normal and pathologic anatomy. This will allow the overlay of multiple types of visual information, including physiologic changes in tissue. Surgical simulation will also change the way that surgeons learn anatomy and surgical techniques. Using the patient's own imaging data, surgeons will first practice the surgery in a realistic environment and explore different surgical corridors.

SUMMARY

Many of the advances in surgery are driven by technologic advances. There has been a revolution in the surgical disciplines since the advent of the endoscope. Over the last decade, a similar revolution has occurred in cranial base surgery, driven by advances in imaging and visualization technologies, dissection instrumentation, hemostatic and reconstructive materials, and neurophysiologic monitoring. The limits of endonasal skull base surgery have not been reached, and it is likely that continued technologic advancement will keep expanding the limits of what can be accomplished endoscopically.

REFERENCES

1. Balzer JR, Kassam AB, Krieger D, et al. Multimodality neurophysiological monitoring during skull base surgery. Skull Base Surg 2001;11(Suppl 1):3.
2. Tabaee A, Anand VK, Fraser JF, et al. Three-dimensional endoscopic pituitary surgery. Neurosurgery 2009;64(5 Suppl 2):288–93 [discussion: 294–5].
3. Samy RN, Krishnamoorthy K, Pensak ML. Use of a novel ultrasonic surgical system for decompression of the facial nerve. Laryngoscope 2007;117(5): 872–5.
4. Kassam A, Snyderman CH, Carrau RL, et al. Endoneurosurgical hemostasis techniques: lessons learned from 400 cases. Neurosurg Focus 2005;19(1):E7.
5. Fischer TH, Connolly R, Thatte HS, et al. Comparison of structural and hemostatic properties of the poly-N-acetyl glucosamine Syvek Patch with products containing chitosan. Microsc Res Tech 2004;63(3):168–74.
6. Stangerup SE, Dommerby H, Siim C, et al. New modification of hot-water irrigation in the treatment of posterior epistaxis. Arch Otolaryngol Head Neck Surg 1999; 125(11):1285.

7. Snyderman CH, Kassam AB, Carrau R, et al. Endoscopic reconstruction of cranial base defects following endonasal skull base surgery. Skull Base 2007;17(1):73–8.
8. Zanation AM, Snyderman CH, Carrau R, et al. Prospective evaluation of the nasoseptal flap for endoscopic reconstruction of high flow intraoperative CSF leaks during endoscopic skull base surgery. Skull Base 2008;18(1):25.
9. Gardner P, Kassam A, Snyderman C, et al. Endoscopic endonasal suturing of reconstruction grafts: a novel application of the U-Clip technology. J Neurosurg 2008;108:395–400.
10. Hadad G, Bassagasteguy L, Carrau RL, et al. A novel reconstructive technique following endoscopic expanded endonasal approaches: vascular pedicle nasoseptal flap. Laryngoscope 2006;116(10):1882–6.

Virtual Simulation in the Surgical World

Marc Gibber, MD[a], Rachel Kaye[b], Marvin P. Fried, MD, PhD[a],*

KEYWORDS

- Surgical simulation • Virtual reality • Medical technology
- Curriculum development • Surgical rehearsal

In light of current technological advances, increased scrutiny of the medical profession, and new directions in medical training, reducing patient risk is of paramount concern, particularly for surgical procedures.

INTRODUCTION TO SIMULATION

Medical-simulator technology is providing students the training media that enable them to achieve proficiency before entering the operating room. This is no surprise given the science of simulation, which is well over 50 years old in other high-risk professions (aviation, nuclear power plants, etc), and has demonstrated the following (Brandon Hall Research News, 2005):

Simulations provide a safe environment in which to make mistakes.
  Some of the best learning comes from assessing your own mistakes.
Well-designed simulations often significantly reduce training time.
  When training on simulators, the focus is on creating the most efficient path for solving a specific problem.
Simulations allow practice of hazardous procedures.
  An example is the ability to practice shutting down a nuclear reactor.
Creating the simulation can help streamline the processes that are being taught.
  Improvements in process are often made when creating simulations.
There can be significant retention of simulation procedures.
  The closer the simulation resembles a learner's actual work environment, the greater the retention.
Simulations allow training to take place without pulling expensive equipment offline.

This work was supported by Award No. W81XWH-05-1-0577 from the Department of Defense, Telemedicine and Technology Research Center (TATRC).

a Department of Otorhinolaryngology—Head and Neck Surgery, Montefiore Medical Center, 3400 Bainbridge Avenue, Bronx, NY, USA
b Albert Einstein College of Medicine, 1300 Morris Park Avenue, Bronx, NY 10461, USA
* Corresponding author.
E-mail address: mfried@montefiore.org (M.P. Fried).

It is prohibitively expensive to pull a $40-million aircraft out of service for training on F-15 aircraft, for example.

Simulations are the best way to transfer expert thinking.

It does this by "modeling" expert behavior in the learning process.

In the medical domain, simulation has become widely accepted over the past 15 years. The medical-simulation validation studies have established that surgical skills honed using a simulator significantly improved trainee performance by decreasing operating times, improving efficiency, and decreasing errors. In short, integration of surgical simulation technologies into the training and education system improves the quality of the graduating surgeon, reduces the time to proficiency, and improves the overall patient safety.[1] The imperative is to develop the devices that can achieve this goal.

The medical profession, academics, authoritative organizations (training, testing, licensing, and certification bodies), and commercial companies have accepted the importance of simulation within the context of a quantitative assessment environment unique to simulators. Evidence of the impact on skills training of using high-fidelity technology that prepares the surgeon before performing the same procedure on a patient has been demonstrated.[2] The impact on patient safety is a priority — mistakes and corrections can be made on a simulator, not on a patient.

Surgery and aviation are sufficiently similar to generate intense interest among surgical educators in the aviation paradigm of training. The obvious training parallel is simulation.[3] Proficiency-based aircrew training has demonstrated that the most effective transfer of training occurred when the student was first proficient in the simulator.[4] With a validated surgical simulator, proficiency criteria can be perfected before permitting the student surgeon to operate on a patient. Therefore, the most pressing need for the near future is to design and validate simulators that train to proficiency within many different specialties.

The American College of Surgeons is interested in promoting surgical simulators by identifying targets for simulation: researching, writing, and implementing the plan for medical-simulation training; and investigating sources of funding.[3] The obstacle to success is bringing the available knowledge and technology together to create devices that are robust, validated, and fluid enough to allow for the potential envisioned. This includes not only training in basic skills but also in the most complex procedures, where performance and judgment are critical. Recreating environments that can be hazardous, again as achieved in flight training, is crucial to the training of a surgeon, with the understanding that patients cannot be placed at risk.

In addition, it is necessary to build a library covering the full range of simple to complex procedures with the many variations that occur from patient to patient. Experiencing the range of procedures from the library along with the busy surgical residency exponentially increases the surgical opportunities within the same given period. For example, just as there has been the traditional medical case of the week to challenge the residents' knowledge and clinical acumen, it will be possible to provide a surgical case of the week on which the trainee can practice.

Surgical rehearsal is an even further development of simulation technology that is achieved because the technology exists to import patient-specific data. As this technology becomes more refined, the surgeon will import the patient-specific image and data, practice the surgical procedure in simulation, and identify critical areas of attention for presentation during the operation. The surgeon will detail the pathology to be addressed (resected, modified, or corrected) and define the areas at risk (such as critical anatomic structures).

A Broader View of Surgical Simulation

High-fidelity virtual reality (VR) simulators have long had an impact on improving the skill level of military and commercial pilots, and they hold similar promise for the medical field. Based on the lessons from aviation training over the past 3 decades, computer-assisted devices have had significant success in augmenting the education and training of surgical residents in several fields.[5–8] VR simulation has already played an introductory role in the training of residents for laparoscopic, gastrointestinal, plastic, ophthalmologic, dermatologic, urologic, and some laryngological proce-dures.[9–16] The efficacy of VR simulation as a teaching tool is clear, but whether it is superior to conventional teaching methods remains uncertain in many instances. Recently, it has been reported that VR training positively influences resident operating room performance and, potentially, safety.[2]

Some early attempts at surgical simulation have met with failure for a number of reasons. First, adequate technology was not available when the concept began to take shape over a decade ago, and the quality of many early surgical simulators was inferior.[6] Second, the science used to evaluate the efficacy of surgical simulators was statistically inadequate and did not measure transfer of training to operating room performance—the ultimate test of a simulator. Finally, the surgical community did not see the value of simulation in all of its variations and applications.

In recent years, as the technology and validation methods have matured and as the surgical community has become more aware of their potential uses, the need for simu-lators to teach, assess, and perhaps even certify surgeons has become apparent.[17] Otolaryngology has taken a leadership role in this pursuit.

Extension to Other Surgical Specialties

While endoscopic techniques have become standard in several other surgical disci-plines, neurosurgeons have only recently started to apply these methods to pituitary and other cranial base lesions.[18–20] Recent studies have compared traditional approaches to the sella turcica using the operating microscope with endoscopic assistance and endoscopic surgery alone.[21,22] No significant difference in outcome was demonstrated in these studies. However, patients operated on with the endo-scopic approach experienced faster recovery, shorter hospital stays, and minimal postoperative discomfort.[18] The two main characteristics of the endoscopic approach, when compared with the standard microsurgical operation, are the use of the endoscope as a unique optical device and the absence of a transsphenoidal retractor.[23] Moreover, the use of an endoscope allows the surgeon to have a clearer picture and better visualization of all the surroundings, inside and outside the sella. There is a trend to minimally invasive neurosurgery, and the concept of training by rehearsal is likely to be generalized in the next years. Specific training is required along with the necessary validation tools to insure safety and efficacy in the treatment of pituitary and other cranial base pathologies.[23–25]

Several surgical procedures in ophthalmology including dacryocystorhinostomy for tear drain obstruction, orbital decompression for thyroid-associated ophthalmop-athy, and optic canal decompression for compressive optic neuropathy have, in recent years, evolved away from transcutaneous and transconjunctival approaches in favor of endoscopic transnasal and transsinus surgical techniques. These tech-niques use the same instrumentation and surgical principals necessary for endo-scopic sinus surgery and require parallel technical and cognitive skills. Currently, clinical training in endoscopic orbital and lacrimal surgical techniques are in the curriculum of fellowship training for the ophthalmic subspecialty of oculoplastic surgery, as defined by the American Society of Ophthalmic Plastic and Reconstructive Surgeons. Traditional transcutaneous and transconjunctival approaches remain in the curriculum of general ophthalmology residency training, and graduates of general ophthalmology training programs are not expected to be proficient in endoscopic surgical techniques.

Preliminary Studies and Rationale

Surgical metrics

In 2002, the Metrics for Technical Skills Conference was convened to create objective measurements that could be assigned to the individual components of an endoscopic sinus surgery procedure.[26] Before this conference, there had been no publication of a classification of errors in endoscopic sinus surgery or a methodology for error occurrence identification and measurement (metrics).

Experts from the fields of medicine, simulation, and education were assembled to identify each error, which were then classified into taxonomy according to the type (technical, cognitive, or combined), and assigned quantifiable measurement units. The final list, as seen in **Box 1**, was approved by consensus. This approach has inculcated a culture of safety into the surgical training program, has been vetted by the American Academy of Otolaryngology-Head and Neck Surgery Foundation and by the American Rhinologic Society. In addition, it has been used as evidence by the American College of Surgeons in their decision to become engaged in surgical simulation as a training modality. For the first time, metrics assigned to an entire surgical procedure may be used as an objective basis for the scoring of surgical skills. The potential of integrating such data into the scoring algorithm of a surgical simulator is apparent.

Validation studies

The process of achieving the goal of objective surgical training and assessment may be intuitively apparent, but it is not arbitrary and requires planned development, evaluation, and implementation.

Validation of proposed virtual simulators is essential in achieving the goal of high stakes assessment (ie, determination of whether a tested individual will advance in their surgical training).[27] The validation studies must be above reproach so that physicians are convinced of the power of simulation as a training tool.[27,28] Only then may surgery accept objective high-stakes assessment.[27]

Numerous validation benchmarks are currently used in the testing literature and, although new to the surgical community, they have been employed in psychology research for more than a century. These benchmarks are recognized as important in creating high-stakes assessment; however, there is currently no mandated requirement for these tests. The process of validating a simulator will be briefly mentioned as it has been extensively discussed elsewhere.[28]

The most subjective validation benchmark tests are used during the initial phases of test construction. These include face validity and content validity and they rely on the input of experts to determine whether the contents of the test are appropriate and whether the test is cohesive. In contrast, concurrent validity is used to compare existing training curriculums or other gold-standard assessment tools to that employed by the simulator. Importantly, discriminant validity focuses on whether the scores generated by the simulator accurately correlates with appropriate factors and is therefore critical in determining whether the simulator is able to stratify the subjects into appropriate skill levels. Predictive validity is commonly the final benchmark test employed. It is essential for determining whether scores on the simulator can accurately predict real skill performance and thus uniquely focuses on clinical outcomes.[28] Predictive validity testing is the most important benchmark test because physicians are concerned with whether simulator training translates to improved skill performance, which in turn imparts improved patient safety.[27]

RESEARCH DESIGN AND METHODS
Software Architecture Development

In order for simulators to operate as patient-specific, they must present the physician with patient-specific realizations of the anatomy and pathology. These realizations should be multisensory and include visualizations and haptic interactions. The visualizations should simulate the physical appearance of anatomy and pathology, including modifications of the visual appearance as the endoscope interacts with the anatomy and pathology. Modifications include the effects of deformations, injections, incisions, resections, ablations, bleeding, and so forth. The haptic interactions should simulate the feel of the instruments as they interact with the anatomy and pathology, and rigid and non-rigid structures, including modifications as the procedure progresses.

Diagnostic images of patients can be used to derive visual and haptic realization of a simulator. This is because CT imagery provides good separation of hard and soft tissue, allowing large cortical bone to be distinguished from the surrounding soft tissue and air passages, while MRI can distinguish various soft tissue types. Simulators that use this technique of image acquisition present the opportunity for patient-specific model generation, introducing the prospect of surgeons being able to practice and rehearse a procedure that is tailored specifically to their patient's anatomy.

Visualization Software Development

It would be remiss in this discussion on visualization not to begin with a caveat. It is wholly recognized that the task of visually emulating all the complex anatomy, tissues, and surgical techniques required for surgery is nontrivial. Albeit daunting, efforts in this direction can provide an advanced level of realism over current techniques, and yield methods that will allow for the continued advancement of the realistic simulation of patient-specific surgeries.

The simulation of realistic bleeding as seen in endoscopic surgeries is particularly difficult. To achieve full realism, a computational fluid dynamic model would be required. This would prove intractable in real time. One current proposed solution is a schematic representation using particle-based methods that exploit the vertex shaders available on the current-generation graphics cards.

The Human Interface Technology Laboratory, at the University of Washington, has developed a video-texture approach[15] to portray bleeding. This technique was developed to support the representation of blood flow during a simulated transurethral resection of the prostate procedure, in which control of excessive bleeding is a concern. Videos were acquired in vitro from an endoscopic view of a physical tube into which red fluid was injected at varying rates and angles. The alpha-mapped video segments were then looped to create a seamless pulsating bleeder which could then be placed (algorithmically or manually) into the virtual prostate anatomy. Trainees were able to handle bleeders either by increasing the fluid flow through the resectoscope or by electrocautery. Similarly, sources of bleeding can be diffuse, which will require broad hemostatic procedures, or focal (eg, specific vessel), which would be an entirely different surgical approach.

Box 1
Taxonomy of errors in endoscopic sinus surgery

Technical

Scope handling

    Scope dirty

    Tool: scope collision

    Contact with wall

    Repetitive scope insertion

    Bleeding obscuring view

    Improper insertion of scope

    Wandering scope unstable

Instrument handling

    Mucosal injury (tissue respect)

    Dissection error

    Past pointing

    Instrument out of view

Controlling field of view

    Lack of perspective

    Image task alignment

Cognitive

Know anatomy

    Misidentifying (anatomic recognition)

    Incomplete examination (leaving out steps)

Know instruments

    Wrong tool choice

    Wrong scope choice

Know procedure sequences

    Task out of sequence

    Omit a step

    Lack of progress

Know procedure technique

    Improper exposure

    Wandering scope: not recognizing target

Not recognizing an injury

    Artery injury

    Bleeding

Combined

Over or under dissection (improper tissue resection)

Injuries

    Orbital injury

    Cranial nerve injury

Lamina papyracea

Cribriform plate injury

Lacrimal system injury

Destabilization of the middle turbinate

Improper location of injection

Rotation (navigation)

From Satava RM, Fried MP. A methodology for objective assessment of errors: an example using an endoscopic sinus surgery simulator. Otolaryngol Clin North Am 35(2002):1289–301.[26]

Curriculum Development

Although closely related, education and training are not the same. Education usually refers to the acquisition of knowledge or information, while training refers to the acquisition of cognitive or psychomotor skills. Most currently available simulators provide training. However, simulators provide only one part of a curriculum, albeit a crucial one. Individuals being prepared to perform a specific procedure need to know what to do, what not to do, how to do it; and this needs to be set in context. As for trainers, they need to know how the trainee is progressing and where he or she is situated on the learning curve. Under the current skill-acquisition paradigm, trainees are required to complete a specified number of procedures or hours of training to be considered competent.[29] In reality, this approach predicts very little other than considerably variable performance levels at the outset of training. Indeed, performance consistency is emerging as one of the best indicators of skill mastery.[30,31]

The paradigm of training to proficiency, or criterion-based training, is the method to address this educational challenge. Flight training is a significant source of inspiration for the implementation of this methodology. Indeed, the longstanding methods used for the training of combat pilots have demonstrated efficiency, and the benefits of their application to surgical education are documented by an increasing number of publications.[3,27,32] There are proven Instructional System Development procedures based on pilot-training design that describe curriculum development in detail[33–35] and can be used to develop a surgical curriculum that incorporates simulation.

This expansion of surgical procedures would require a reexamination of the Surgical Essential Competencies (SECs) required for successful completion of each identified procedure. SECs are the knowledge and skills that a specialist exhibits routinely to successfully accomplish specified surgical procedures. SECs are a foundation construct for developing a robust curriculum. This competency-based approach also provides a level of detail and analysis necessary to address the complexity of operations. Application of this approach aids in reducing the learning curve for the entry-level surgeon. This approach changes mission readiness from being defined in terms of number of hours and surgeries observed and accomplished, into a definition in terms of required level of performance under real-world conditions, in specific surgical contexts (proficiency). Competencies can be captured over the range of known normal, abnormal, and emergency conditions. SECs are organized to define a starting point, purpose, and end point for a given procedure. Mission scenarios can be defined for the specific surgical contexts of each specialty, which represent the performance requirements, operational conditions, and standards of performance outcomes. A competency-based approach helps optimize the already successful residency using advanced simulation. The curriculum would also have broad application for medical student education and broad specialty-wide evaluation.

Surgical Rehearsal

Surgical rehearsal is defined as simulated patient-specific run-through by the operating surgeon before performance of the actual operation. Surgical rehearsal input is correlated with the surgical navigation system to provide the surgeon critical focal points, with annotations to follow, during the operation. High-end simulation provides the scene presentation and haptic feedback in which the surgeon will experience VR. From the surgeon's perspective, the difference between surgical rehearsal and operational performance will be the shift to a live patient.

From the inception of the first VR system in endoscopic surgery, the vision has been for the surgeon to rehearse the surgical procedure before carrying it out on the patient. This vision comes directly from the aviation industry where pilots are trained on high-fidelity simulators before they fly a real aircraft. Marescaux, and colleagues,[36] demonstrated that it was possible to download patient-specific data that can provide good guides as to how surgery should be completed. The visualization technology now exists for accurate surgical rehearsal, a technique that carries the goals of reduced variability in performance and decreased procedure time. This is achievable in temporal bone surgery. Achieving these goals will translate into improved patient safety.

SUMMARY

The development of simulation-training technology together with a universal curriculum for educational implementation of the technology constitutes the future of successful surgical care in this country and worldwide. Medical students and surgical residents will be able, and mandated, to develop procedural skills in a life-like and no-risk environment where emphasis is placed on education rather than treatment, and on the student rather than a patient. Curriculum design will include basic procedures deemed generally applicable in surgical fields across the board, in addition to field-specific procedures and operating room scenarios. The curriculum will be designed as both a means of imbuing all trainees with these universal and field-specific skills, and as a means of identifying elements of procedure with which they have particular difficulty. There will be additional skill-specific training programs designed for those exhibiting poor performance in one particular procedure or skill.

Furthermore, the development of a library of simple and complex procedural data will allow for training in the same procedure with various deviations in anatomy and pathology. The trainees will be exposed to varying versions of the same procedure, thereby allowing for diversification of experience and ability. Only upon achievement that meets established benchmarks of proficiency will trainees be validated as suitable for live surgical activity. In this way, surgical residents can obtain extensive operating room experience and develop comprehensive surgical skills before working on a live patient. Resident-specific weaknesses will have been addressed, and a considerable degree of comfort in various procedures will have been reached.

There is already support from the surgical governing and regulation agencies (American College of Surgeons, American Academy of Otolaryngology—Head and Neck Surgery, American Board of Otolaryngology, etc). Application to military medicine is apparent also. Participation by commercial companies will guarantee that there will be real deliverables—simulators capable of training and mission rehearsal, and a digital library of challenging cases for residents to practice. The open platform that will be fashioned by this application will guarantee access to the products of this research to the entire scientific community.

REFERENCES

1. Gallagher, AG. VR to OR. In: Medicine Meets Virtual Reality Conference (MMVR 11). 2003, Newport Beach, CA.
2. Seymour NE, Gallagher AG, Roman SA, et al. Virtual reality training improves operating room performance: results of a randomized, double-blinded study. Ann Surg 2002;236(4):458–63 [discussion: 463–4].
3. McGreevy JM. The aviation paradigm and surgical education. J Am Coll Surg 2005;201(1):110–7.
4. Bills CG, Spears WD. Design guide for device-based aircrew training. Information for designers of instructional systems. AF Handbook 36-2235. Washington, DC: Department of the Air Force; 1993. p. 7.
5. O'Toole RV, Playter RR, Krummel TM, et al. Measuring and developing suturing technique with a virtual reality surgical simulator. J Am Coll Surg 1999;189(1): 114–27.
6. Satava RM. Virtual reality surgical simulator. The first steps. Surg Endosc 1993; 7(3):203–5.
7. Gorman PJ, Meier AH, Krummel TM. Computer-assisted training and learning in surgery. Comput Aided Surg 2000;5(2):120–30.
8. McGovern KT. Applications of virtual reality to surgery. BMJ 1994;308(6936): 1054–5.
9. Satava RM. Virtual endoscopy: diagnosis using 3-D visualization and virtual representation. Surg Endosc 1996;10(2):173–4.
10. Baillie J, Evangelou H, Jowell P, et al. The future of endoscopy simulation: a Duke perspective. Endoscopy 1992;24(Suppl 2):542–3.
11. Fried MP, Moharir VM, Shinmoto H, et al. Virtual laryngoscopy. Ann Otol Rhinol Laryngol 1999;108(3):221–6.
12. Peugnet F, Dubois P, Rouland JF. Virtual reality versus conventional training in retinal photocoagulation: a first clinical assessment. Comput Aided Surg 1998; 3(1):20–6.
13. Gladstone HB, Raugi GJ, Berg D, et al. Virtual reality for dermatologic surgery: virtually a reality in the 21st century. J Am Acad Dermatol 2000;42(1 Pt 1):106–12.
14. Berg D, Raugi G, Gladstone H, et al. Virtual reality simulators for dermatologic surgery: measuring their validity as a teaching tool. Dermatol Surg 2001;27(4): 370–4.
15. Oppenheimer P, Gupta A, Weghorst S, et al. The representation of blood flow in endourologic surgical simulations. Stud Health Technol Inform 2001;81:365–71.
16. Edmond CV Jr, Heskamp D, Sluis D, et al. ENT endoscopic surgical training simulator. Stud Health Technol Inform 1997;39:518–28.
17. Gallagher AG, Ritter EM, Champion H, et al. Virtual reality simulation for the operating room: proficiency-based training as a paradigm shift in surgical skills training. Ann Surg 2005;241(2):364–72.
18. Jho HD, Alfieri A. Endoscopic endonasal pituitary surgery: evolution of surgical technique and equipment in 150 operations. Minim Invasive Neurosurg 2001; 44(1):1–12.
19. Kassam A, Snyderman CH, Mintz A, et al. Expanded endonasal approach: the rostrocaudal axis. Part I. *Crista galli* to the *sella turcica*. Neurosurg Focus 2005; 19(1):E3.

20. Kassam A, Snyderman CH, Mintz A, et al. Expanded endonasal approach: the rostrocaudal axis. Part II. Posterior clinoids to the foramen magnum. Neurosurg Focus 2005;19(1):E4.
21. Jho HD. Endoscopic pituitary surgery. Pituitary 1999;2(2):139–54.
22. Jho HD, Alfieri A. Endoscopic transsphenoidal pituitary surgery: various surgical techniques and recommended steps for procedural transition. Br J Neurosurg 2000;14(5):432–40.
23. Cappabianca P, Cavallo LM, Esposito F, et al. Endoscopic endonasal trans-sphenoidal surgery: procedure, endoscopic equipment and instrumentation. Childs Nerv Syst 2004;20(11–12):796–801.
24. Rudnik A, Zawadzki T, Wojtacha M, et al. Endoscopic transnasal trans-sphenoidal treatment of pathology of the sellar region. Minim Invasive Neurosurg 2005;48(2):101–7.
25. de Divitiis E, Cappabianca P. Endoscopic pituitary surgery. Tuttlingen (Germany): Endo-Press; 2005.
26. Satava RM, Fried MP. A methodology for objective assessment of errors: an example using an endoscopic sinus surgery simulator. Otolaryngol Clin North Am 2002;35(6):1289–301.
27. Fried MP, Gallagher AG, Satava RM. Training to proficiency: aircraft to OR. Arch Otolaryngol Head Neck Surg 2004;130(10):1145–6.
28. Gallagher AG, Ritter EM, Satava RM. Fundamental principles of validation, and reliability: rigorous science for the assessment of surgical education and training. Surg Endosc 2003;17(10):1525–9 [Epub 2003 Sep 19].
29. Cass OW. Training to competence in gastrointestinal endoscopy: a plea for continuous measuring of objective end points. Endoscopy 1999;31(9):751–4.
30. Gallagher AG, Richie K, McClure N, et al. Objective psychomotor skills assessment of experienced, junior, and novice laparoscopists with virtual reality. World J Surg 2001;25(11):1478–83.
31. Gallagher AG, Satava RM. Virtual reality as a metric for the assessment of laparoscopic psychomotor skills. Learning curves and reliability measures. Surg Endosc 2002;16(12):1746–52.
32. Muller MH. How does aviation find the ideal pilot? Suitability testing: applicability to surgery? Methods for determining basic occupational suitability. Zentralbl Chir 1999;124(10):889–94.
33. Schufletowski FW. Information for designers of instructional systems—ISD executive summary for commanders and managers. AF Handbook 36-2235. Washington, DC: Department of the Air Force; 2002. p.1.
34. Bills CG, D Devol. How F-16 MTC team achieved operational training capability. In: Interservice/Industry Training, Simulation, and Education Conference (I/ITSEC), 2003.
35. Bills CG. Instructional system development (ISD) planning for large development projects. In: Performance-based instructional systems design conference. International Society for Performance Improvement (ISPI); 2004.
36. Marescaux J, Clément JM, Tassetti V, et al. Virtual reality applied to hepatic surgery simulation: the next revolution. Ann Surg 1998;228(5):627–34.

Cranial-Base Repair Using Endoscopic Laser Welding

Benjamin S. Bleier, MD[a], James N. Palmer, MD[b],*

KEYWORDS

• Laser • Tissue welding • Skull-base reconstruction
• Cerebrospinal fluid leak repair • Solder
• Chromophore

The field of endoscopic cranial-base surgery has undergone significant evolution in the past decade, fueled largely by advances in imaging and instrumentation. While the limits of these approaches have yet to be reached, difficulties in reconstructing the resultant defects have become significant obstacles. Successful reconstruction requires a technique that recapitulates the complex morphology of the cranial base while simultaneously withstanding the hydrostatic forces exerted by the cerebrospinal fluid compartment. Current strategies have evolved around the fundamental limitations of access in endoscopic approaches and thus represent a departure from the principles of surgical closure in an open field. In place of meticulous tissue apposition and watertight suture lines, surgeons are limited to multilayer grafting and the liberal application of relatively weak biologic glues, which often obscure the defect, thereby impairing the intraoperative assessment of the closure. These techniques may require prolonged nasal packing and lumbar drain placement to further support the repair in the immediate postoperative period. Despite these limitations, the low-pressure profile of cerebrospinal fluid coupled with the dense vascularity of the dura and mucosa allow for robust wound healing leading to successful closure in the vast majority of cases. The recent introduction of vascularized rotational flaps has further improved outcomes in several series. However, there remains an overall 10% failure rate, which may increase as skull-base approaches continue to expand. These problems have catalyzed a search for a repair method that can be applied endoscopically

Some of the data described in the article were obtained with the support of the 2007 American Rhinologic Society Resident Research Grant entitled "In Vivo Laser Tissue Welding in the Rabbit Paranasal Sinus."

[a] Department of Otorhinolaryngology—Head and Neck Surgery, University of Pennsylvania School of Medicine, 1324 Pinewood Road, Villanova, Philadelphia, PA 19085, USA
[b] Division of Rhinology, Department of Otorhinolaryngology—Head and Neck Surgery, University of Pennsylvania School of Medicine, 3400 Spruce Street, Philadelphia, PA 19104, USA
* Corresponding author.
E-mail address: james.palmer@uphs.upenn.edu (J.N. Palmer).

oto.theclinics.com

and is capable of producing instant, watertight tissue bonds. Laser tissue welding has been advanced as one such technology that may satisfy these criteria and further reduce the morbidity and failure rate of cranial-base reconstruction.

Since their invention in the late 1950s, lasers have been successfully used in a variety of medical fields as both diagnostic and therapeutic instruments. As early as 1960, the potential for use of lasers in tissue adhesion was recognized. In 1962, Sigel and Acevado[1] were the first to report the potential of thermal energy in tissue adhesion by using high-frequency electric current to create an end-to-side portocaval shunt in a canine model. Yahr and Strully[2] adapted this concept to light energy and are credited with the first description of laser tissue welding for vascular anastomosis. The early work in laser tissue welding primarily used Nd:YAG (neodymium:yttrium-aluminum-garnet) systems.[3] As technology advanced, a wider variety of laser systems entered the clinical armamentarium, including the argon, the carbon dioxide, and the diode laser, which allowed researchers to tailor the laser wavelength and depth of penetration to the tissue being studied.[4] While these initial reports demonstrated the potential of laser tissue welding, in vivo applications were limited by suboptimal wound tensile strength and complications related to thermal leakage to surrounding healthy tissues.

A critical advance in laser tissue welding came over the last 2 decades with the introduction of biologic solder materials coupled with wavelength-specific chromophores, such as indocyanine green, fluorescein, and carbon black.[4,5] These materials allowed for target-specific laser energy absorption and reduced the degree of collateral thermal leakage.[6] Histologic analysis of wounds repaired using a biologic solder demonstrated that the direct thermal injury was restricted to the top 20 μm of the solder without any evidence of underlying tissue injury.[6,7] This evidence of good target-specific characteristics is further supported by a study in an esophageal fistula model in which no thermal injury was noted in the esophageal mucosa following laser-assisted closure using an albumin-based solder.[8] The chromophore provides a secondary benefit by providing a predictable color change, which established an objective basis of gauging adequacy of lasing.[9] Some investigators have described a computer-based thermal feedback system to further define the lasing end point.[6] However, its practical utility in light of the negligible thermal effect previously described remains to be seen.

Multiple combinations of biologic solders have been described, including collagen- and fibrin-based formulations. However, the most promising results have been reported using an albumin-based solution coupled with indocyanine green dye and hyaluronic acid.[10] The use of biologic solders has also been shown to promote native wound-healing mechanisms. In contrast to the granulomatous inflammatory response seen with suture material, the lased solder provides a nonimmunogenic scaffold.[9] This coagulum is gradually absorbed during the normal wound-healing process[11,12] with minimal disruption of elastic fibers[13] and a similar collagen density seen with traditional wound-closure techniques.[14] A study in porcine dura reported integration of vascular and fibrous tissue into the repair within a week, demonstrating that normal wound healing is unimpeded by the solder-enhanced weld.[15]

While a considerable amount of research has gone into optimizing laser-welding techniques in a variety of animal models, the precise mechanism of tissue bonding has yet to be fully explained. Most investigators agree that the application of laser energy results in a restructuring of the extracellular matrix with resultant interactions of native tissue proteins, including collagen interdigitation, and noncovalent laminin and entactin bonding.[7,9,16] Murray and colleagues[17] demonstrated a decrease in both a 235-kd guanidine-extractable protein and type VI collagen with a concomitant rise in protein aggregates with noncollagenous domains, suggesting that fibronectin is also involved. Although these studies have contributed to our grasp of the mechanism of laser tissue welding, a complete understanding remains confounded by multiple variables, including laser wavelength, tissue-specific energy absorption, and the use of a variety of solder and chromophore formulations.[4]

Laser tissue welding using an albumin-based solder has been studied in a variety of tissues, including blood vessels, gut, nerves, skin, dura, bladder, and urethra.[14] Despite our incomplete understanding of the mechanism, these studies have consistently confirmed that it is an efficacious method of tissue bonding capable of creating instant welds with significant tensile strength and high leak pressures. Barrieras and colleagues[14] compared laser-welded pyeloplasty using an albumin/fibrin solder to both traditional suture and fibrin glue repair. This study found an immediate increase in anastomotic leak pressure using a laser weld over both suture and fibrin glue (37.2 ± 1.1 mm Hg as compared with 12.8 ± 4.0 mm Hg and 2.6 ± 1.1 mm Hg, respectively). In 1996, Foyt and colleagues[7] performed one of the first ex vivo studies examining the utility of laser tissue welding in a head and neck application. This group looked at primary human cadaveric dural closure using an albumin/indocyanine green dye mixture. They reported a leak pressure of 26.2 ± 3.7 mm Hg with the laser closure as compared with 9.4 ± 1.7 mm Hg in the suture group. These studies underscore the fact that the efficacy of the weld depends on both the laser/solder combination as well as the tissue being addressed. The spectral absorption characteristics, extracellular matrix composition, and tensile properties of the underlying tissue all play an important role in the behavior of the lased coagulum. As a result, the validation of laser tissue welding as a reconstructive technique mandates preclinical studies that use a single laser/solder platform and address the tissues that are specifically relevant to cranial-base repair. While weld strength is the primary determinant of the utility of laser tissue welding, these studies must also address the prospective effects on wound healing as well as the risk of thermal injury inherent to the use of lasers in any clinical application.

The 808-nm diode laser coupled with a solder based on 42% human albumin, indocyanine green, and hyaluronic acid has been the most extensively studied in both animal and clinical trials and has thus become the basis of our investigations. In our initial study, our group demonstrated that laser tissue welding is capable of producing in sheep septal mucosa and periosteum burst strengths that were significantly higher than those of suture repair (mucosa: 34.88 ± 3.49 mm Hg versus 17.06 ± 1.83 mm Hg, P = .0001; periosteum: 30.02 ± 2.23 mm Hg versus 24.12 ± 0.71 mm Hg, $P<.0001$) (**Fig. 1**).[18] These data were used to establish an animal model in the New Zealand white rabbit to analyze the prospective behavior of these welds in the repair of a dorsal maxillary sinusotomy.[19] This study found that laser welding was capable of achieving an immediate burst strength over four times that of normal human intracranial pressure. The strength of these bonds increased over the first 2 weeks and was noted to converge with those of an open wound left to heal by secondary intention by postoperative day 15 (**Fig. 2**). This offers an interesting insight into the natural history of these wounds in a clinical setting, where it appears that native scarring and fibrosis alone are capable of sealing these defects within several weeks, confirming that efforts should be focused on preventing early repair failures. The other key finding of this study was that no thermal injury was noted to the surrounding tissues or underlying sinus mucosa (**Fig. 3**). The lack of collateral thermal injury represents a critical attribute of laser tissue welding, especially when considering the proximity of these repairs to critical neurovascular structures. While not formally reported, the investigators also noted that, at the low irradiances required to effect these welds, the laser shows no clinical effect when applied directly to the tissue.

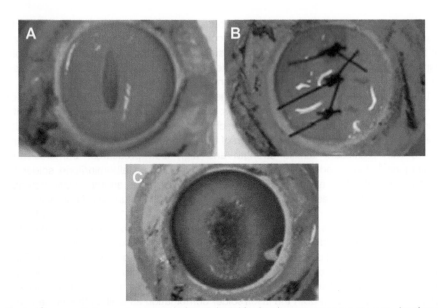

Fig. 1. Sheep septal mucosa suspended in a closed hydraulic manometry system under three experimental conditions: (A) Open wound. (B) Interrupted suture closure. (C) Laser welded closure. (*From* Bleier BS, Palmer JN, Sparano AM, et al. Laser assisted cerebrospinal fluid leak repair: an animal model to test feasibility. Otolaryngol Head Neck Surg 2007;137(5):810–4.)

Despite the success of these animal studies, clinical data are still required to determine the safety and technical feasibility of this technique in an operative field. Kirsch and colleagues[9] reported a clinical trial using the same laser/solder platform in human ureteroplasty and noted significantly higher intraoperative leak threshold pressures in laser solder–reinforced microsutured incision lines than in suture alone (94.2 ± 24.2 mm Hg versus 20.0 ± 2.9 mm Hg, $P<.001$) in a study of 10 patients. While these data are encouraging, unique challenges to the endoscopic application of this technique must still be overcome.

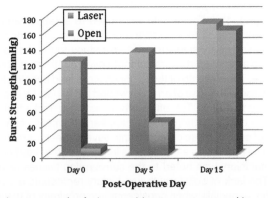

Fig. 2. Prospective burst strength of a laser weld versus open wound in a rabbit dorsal maxillary sinusotomy model. Laser welds on postoperative day 0 and 5 are significantly stronger than the open wound ($P<.05$). (*Data from* Bleier BS, Palmer JN, Gratton MA, et al. Laser tissue welding in the rabbit maxillary sinus. Am J Rhinol 2008;22(6):625–8.)

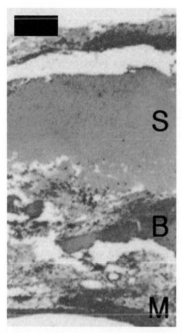

Fig. 3. Hemotoxylin and eosin image of lased solder coagulum (S) overlying the bone (B) and mucosa (M) of the dorsal maxillary sinusotomy with negligible collateral thermal injury (bar represents 100 μm).

While the 808-nm diode laser–42% human albumin solder combination has been shown to be safe and efficacious, the clinical success of endoscopic laser welding will likely hinge on the viscoelastic properties of the solder itself. In a low-viscosity formulation, the solder will tend to run off the skull base toward the dependent areas of the field and be diluted by blood and irrigation. These formulations often have a high water content requiring a longer lasing time to heat the solution to the temperature required for protein denaturation. This is not only inconvenient but also prolongs the thermal exposure of the surrounding tissue. Conversely, high-viscosity solutions and solids are difficult to apply endoscopically and are less likely to interpolate themselves into the interstices of the wound, resulting in gaps, which can lead to repair failure. Novel solder formulations are currently being developed that seek to incorporate the benefits of both low- and high-viscosity solutions. However, their safety and thermal profiles must be clearly established before their clinical use.

SUMMARY

Reconstruction of the cranial base remains a significant challenge to the progress of endoscopic skull-base surgery. Laser tissue welding offers the potential of creating instant, watertight repairs that may obviate the need for postoperative nasal packing and lumbar drain placement. While this technology appears promising in animal studies, clinical safety parameters must be fully elaborated before its incorporation into the clinical armamentarium. In addition to safety issues, issues pertaining specifically to endoscopic laser welding, including solder viscosity, must be addressed to ensure intra- and interoperator reproducibility. While laser tissue welding remains an experimental technique, its future in the field on endoscopic skull-base surgery remains bright.

REFERENCES

1. Sigel B, Acevado FJ. Vein anastomosis by electrocoaptive union. Surg Forum 1962;13:233–5.
2. Yahr WZ, Strully KJ. Blood vessel anastamosis by laser and other biomedical applications. J Assoc Adv Med Instrum 1966;(1):28–31.
3. Flock ST, Marchitto KS. Progress towards seamless tissue fusion for wound closure. Otolaryngol Clin North Am 2005;38(2):295–305.
4. Talmor M, Bleustein CB, Poppas DP. Laser tissue welding: a biotechnological advance for the future. Arch Facial Plast Surg 2001;3(3):207–13.
5. Oz MC, Johnson JP, Parangi S, et al. Tissue soldering by use of indocyanine green dye-enhanced fibrinogen with the near infrared diode laser. J Vasc Surg 1990;11(5):718–25.
6. Gil Z, Shaham A, Vasilyev T, et al. Novel laser tissue-soldering technique for dural reconstruction. J Neurosurg 2005;103(1):87–91.
7. Foyt D, Johnson JP, Kirsch AJ, et al. Dural closure with laser tissue welding. Otolaryngol Head Neck Surg 1996;115(6):513–8.
8. Bleier BS, Gratton MA, Leibowitz JM, et al. Laser welded endoscopic endoluminal repair of iatrogenic esophageal perforation: an animal model. Otolaryngol Head Neck Surg 2008;139(5):713–7.
9. Kirsch AJ, Miller MI, Hensle TW, et al. Laser tissue soldering in urinary tract reconstruction: first human experience. Urology 1995;46(2):261–6.
10. Wright EJ, Poppas DP. Effect of laser wavelength and protein solder concentration on acute tissue repair using laser welding: initial results in a canine ureter model. Tech Urol 1997;3(3):176–81.
11. Lauto A, Kerman I, Ohebshalon M, et al. Two-layer film as a laser soldering biomaterial. Lasers Surg Med 1999;25(3):250–6.
12. Lauto A, Trickett R, Malik R, et al. Laser-activated solid protein bands for peripheral nerve repair: an vivo study. Lasers Surg Med 1997;21(2):134–41.
13. Abergel RP, Lyons R, Dwyer R, et al. Use of lasers for closure of cutaneous wounds: experience with Nd:YAG, argon and CO2 lasers. J Dermatol Surg Oncol 1986;12(11):1181–5.
14. Barrieras D, Reddy PP, McLorie GA, et al. Lessons learned from laser tissue soldering and fibrin glue pyeloplasty in an in vivo porcine model. J Urol 2000; 164(3 Pt 2):1106–10.
15. Tachibana E, Saito K, Fukuta K, et al. Evaluation of the healing process after dural reconstruction achieved using a free fascial graft. J Neurosurg 2002;96(2):280–6.
16. Helmsworth TF, Wright CB, Scheffter SM, et al. Molecular surgery of the basement membrane by the argon laser. Lasers Surg Med 1990;10(6):576–83.
17. Murray LW, Su L, Kopchok GE, et al. Crosslinking of extracellular matrix proteins: a preliminary report on a possible mechanism of argon laser welding. Lasers Surg Med 1989;9(5):490–6.
18. Bleier BS, Palmer JN, Sparano AM, et al. Laser assisted cerebrospinal fluid leak repair: an animal model to test feasibility. Otolaryngol Head Neck Surg 2007; 137(5):810–4.
19. Bleier BS, Palmer JN, Gratton MA, et al. Laser tissue welding in the rabbit maxillary sinus. Am J Rhinol 2008;22(6):625–8.

Index

Note: Page numbers of article titles are in **boldface** type.

Otolaryngol Clin N Am 42 (2009) 907–913
doi:10.1016/S0030-6665(09)00156-X
0030-6665/09/$ – see front matter © 2009 Elsevier Inc. All rights reserved.

United States Postal Service

Statement of Ownership, Management, and Circulation
(All Periodicals Publications Except Requestor Publications)

1. Publication Title	2. Publication Number	3. Filing Date
Otolaryngologic Clinics of North America	4 6 6 - 5 5 5 0	9/15/09

4. Issue Frequency	5. Number of Issues Published Annually	6. Annual Subscription Price
Feb, Apr, Jun, Aug, Oct, Dec	6	$264.00

7. Complete Mailing Address of Known Office of Publication (Not printer) (Street, city, county, state, and ZIP+4®)

Elsevier Inc.
360 Park Avenue South
New York, NY 10010-1710

Contact Person
Stephen Bushing
Telephone (Include area code)
215-239-3688

8. Complete Mailing Address of Headquarters or General Business Office of Publisher (Not printer)

Elsevier Inc., 360 Park Avenue South, New York, NY 10010-1710

9. Full Names and Complete Mailing Addresses of Publisher, Editor, and Managing Editor (Do not leave blank)

Publisher (Name and complete mailing address)

John Schrefer, Elsevier, Inc., 1600 John F. Kennedy Blvd. Suite 1800, Philadelphia, PA 19103-2899

Editor (Name and complete mailing address)

Joanne Husovski, Elsevier, Inc., 1600 John F. Kennedy Blvd. Suite 1800, Philadelphia, PA 19103-2899

Managing Editor (Name and complete mailing address)

Catherine Bewick, Elsevier, Inc., 1600 John F. Kennedy Blvd. Suite 1800, Philadelphia, PA 19103-2899

10. Owner (Do not leave blank. If the publication is owned by a corporation, give the name and address of the corporation immediately followed by the names and addresses of all stockholders owning or holding 1 percent or more of the total amount of stock. If not owned by a corporation, give the names and addresses of the individual owners. If owned by a partnership or other unincorporated firm, give its name and address as well as those of each individual owner. If the publication is published by a nonprofit organization, give its name and address.)

Full Name	Complete Mailing Address
Wholly owned subsidiary of	4520 East-West Highway
Reed/Elsevier, US holdings	Bethesda, MD 20814

11. Known Bondholders, Mortgagees, and Other Security Holders Owning or Holding 1 Percent or More of Total Amount of Bonds, Mortgages, or Other Securities. If none, check box. ☐ None

Full Name	Complete Mailing Address
N/A	

12. Tax Status (For completion by nonprofit organizations authorized to mail at nonprofit rates) (Check one)
The purpose, function, and nonprofit status of this organization and the exempt status for federal income tax purposes:
☐ Has Not Changed During Preceding 12 Months
☐ Has Changed During Preceding 12 Months (Publisher must submit explanation of change with this statement)

PS Form 3526, September 2007 (Page 1 of 3 (Instructions Page 3)) PSN 7530-01-000-9931 PRIVACY NOTICE. See our Privacy policy in www.usps.com

13. Publication Title	14. Issue Date for Circulation Data Below
Otolaryngologic Clinics of North America	June 2009

15. Extent and Nature of Circulation		Average No. Copies Each Issue During Preceding 12 Months	No. Copies of Single Issue Published Nearest to Filing Date
a. Total Number of Copies (Net press run)		2650	2298
b. Paid Circulation (By Mail and Outside the Mail)	(1) Mailed Outside-County Paid Subscriptions Stated on PS Form 3541. (Include paid distribution above nominal rate, advertiser's proof copies, and exchange copies)	1129	1074
	(2) Mailed In-County Paid Subscriptions Stated on PS Form 3541 (Include paid distribution above nominal rate, advertiser's proof copies, and exchange copies)		
	(3) Paid Distribution Outside the Mails Including Sales Through Dealers and Carriers, Street Vendors, Counter Sales, and Other Paid Distribution Outside USPS®	768	713
	(4) Paid Distribution by Other Classes Mailed Through the USPS (e.g. First-Class Mail®)		
c. Total Paid Distribution (Sum of 15b (1), (2), (3), and (4))	▶	1897	1787
d. Free or Nominal Rate Distribution (By Mail and Outside the Mail)	(1) Free or Nominal Rate Outside-County Copies Included on PS Form 3541	103	76
	(2) Free or Nominal Rate In-County Copies Included on PS Form 3541		
	(3) Free or Nominal Rate Copies Mailed at Other Classes Through the USPS (e.g. First-Class Mail)		
	(4) Free or Nominal Rate Distribution Outside the Mail (Carriers or other means)		
e. Total Free or Nominal Rate Distribution (Sum of 15d (1), (2), (3) and (4))	▶	103	76
f. Total Distribution (Sum of 15c and 15e)	▶	2000	1863
g. Copies not Distributed (See instructions to publishers #4 (page #3))	▶	650	435
h. Total (Sum of 15f and g)	▶	2650	2298
i. Percent Paid (15c divided by 15f times 100)		94.85%	95.92%

16. Publication of Statement of Ownership
☐ If the publication is a general publication, publication of this statement is required. Will be printed in the October 2009 issue of this publication. ☐ Publication not required.

17. Signature and Title of Editor, Publisher, Business Manager, or Owner

Stephen R. Bushing
Stephen R. Bushing – Subscription Services Coordinator

Date September 15, 2009

I certify that all information furnished on this form is true and complete. I understand that anyone who furnishes false or misleading information on this form or who omits material or information requested on the form may be subject to criminal sanctions (including fines and imprisonment) and/or civil sanctions (including civil penalties).

PS Form 3526, September 2007 (Page 2 of 3)

Moving?

Make sure your subscription moves with you!

To notify us of your new address, find your **Clinics Account Number** (located on your mailing label above your name), and contact customer service at:

Email: journalscustomerservice-usa@elsevier.com

800-654-2452 (subscribers in the U.S. & Canada)
314-447-8871 (subscribers outside of the U.S. & Canada)

Fax number: 314-447-8029

Elsevier Health Sciences Division
Subscription Customer Service
3251 Riverport Lane
Maryland Heights, MO 63043

*To ensure uninterrupted delivery of your subscription,
please notify us at least 4 weeks in advance of move.

Printed and bound by CPI Group (UK) Ltd, Croydon, CR0 4YY

03/10/2024

01040464-0016